OXFORD MEDICAL PU

Psychiatry

Key questions answered

More Key questions answered:

Clinical Medicine
Wai-Ching Leung

Endocrinology
John Laycock and Peter Wise

Paediatrics
Jonathan Round

Psychiatry
Polash Shajahan, Alan Doris, Deborah Nelson, and Mark Taylor

Psychiatry
Key questions answered

Polash Shajahan

Clinical Scientist and Honorary Specialist Registrar, MRC Brain Metabolism Unit, Royal Edinburgh Hospital, Edinburgh

Alan Doris

Clinical Scientist and Honorary Specialist Registrar, MRC Brain Metabolism Unit, Royal Edinburgh Hospital, Edinburgh

Deborah Nelson

Specialist Registrar, Royal Edinburgh Hospital, Edinburgh

Mark Taylor

Senior Registrar, Royal Edinburgh Hospital, Edinburgh

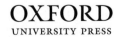

OXFORD

UNIVERSITY PRESS

OXFORD

UNIVERSITY PRESS

Great Clarendon Street, Oxford OX2 6DP

Oxford University Press is a department of the University of Oxford
and furthers the University's aim of excellence in research, scholarship,
and education by publishing worldwide in

Oxford New York

Athens Auckland Bangkok Bogotá Buenos Aires Calcutta
Cape Town Chennai Dar es Salaam Delhi Florence Hong Kong Istanbul
Karachi Kuala Lumpur Madrid Melbourne Mexico City Mumbai
Nairobi Paris São Paulo Singapore Taipei Tokyo Toronto Warsaw
and associated companies in Berlin Ibadan

Oxford is a registered trade mark of Oxford University Press

Published in the United States
by Oxford University Press Inc., New York

A catalogue record for this book is available from the British Library

Library of Congress Cataloging in Publication Data
(Data applied for)

ISBN 0 19 263033 4 (Pbk)

Typeset by
Footnote Graphics, Warminster, Wilts

Printed in Great Britain on acid free paper by
Biddles Ltd., Guildford, Surrey

Contents

Introduction

The written examination for the membership of the Royal College of Psychiatrists (MRCPsych) consists of an essay paper, a critical review paper, and two multiple choice papers. Each of these aspects of the exam tests different abilities in the candidate. This book relates specifically to how to maximize the chances of success in the MCQ papers.

The MCQ papers have been a central part of the Royal College of Psychiatrists' membership examination for many years and are likely to continue to be so in the future. They are the main test of the candidate's factual knowledge in both basic science and clinical topics. Much of the popularity of the MCQ in postgraduate examinations is due to the objectivity of the marking system.

The MRCPsych exam

Although this text can be used in preparation for other psychiatric examinations it is primarily aimed at the MRCPsych. Possession of the MRCPsych is essential for progression to higher training in psychiatry in the UK and hence is a prerequisite for specialist status in psychiatry in Britain (and thus also Europe).

The MRCPsych exam is divided into two parts. This book is intended as preparation for the Part II, which is generally considered a more wide-ranging and searching test than the Part I exam. Eligibility for entrance into the Part II MRCPsych is determined by successful completion of the Part I examination, and ongoing satisfactory training in a recognized scheme. Entrance into the Part II exam should be discussed with your local clinical tutor, and details about eligibility as well as other exam essentials are obtainable from the Royal College of Psychiatry examinations department:

Examinations Department
Royal College of Psychiatrists
17 Belgrave Square
London SW1 X8PG, UK
Telephone (+44) 0171 235 2351

General preparation for MRCPsych Part II

Attempting Part II of the MRCPsych is a major undertaking that will have a large impact on your life. Before applying to sit the exam it is wise to consider if now is the right time for you. If there are foreseeable major life events around the time of the exam it may be better to delay until a more suitable time and save yourself a lot of time, money, and anguish. Your clinical tutor should be able to give helpful advice in this regard.

It is essential to contact the Examinations Department of the College well in advance of the closing date for applications to ensure that all necessary paperwork is completed in good time.

Preparation for the exam is a process that proceeds throughout basic training in psychiatry; however, more focused work is required in the months leading up to the exam to ensure success. We feel that an absolute minimum of time required for revision prior to the exam is 3 months.

Both the MCQ papers—Basic Science and Clinical—comprise 50 individual items in 5 parts. Both papers are negatively marked. It is worth remembering that there is no absolute pass mark in the MCQ papers, and that each MCQ paper is essentially a competitive test with about 40–45% of the cohort taking the paper being adjudged successful.

How to study

It is advisable that your study for the exam should proceed in a reasonably organized fashion with a programme of work drawn up and revised regularly as time passes. Setting aside regular protected time that is dedicated to study is most useful, ensuring that the time spent studying is in manageable chunks so that you do not become excessively fatigued or stale. If you are drawing up a work schedule, remember to timetable in periods of recreation and rest as this will make the overall task easier and probably also enhance learning (as long as these periods are not excessive!).

Candidates necessarily do most of their revision on their own, though the use of study groups of one form or another is to be recommended. Studying with colleagues prevents the individual candidate from becoming side-tracked into one particular area of study and neglecting others. Many candidates find that some group revision can be helpful and supportive, particularly when the study group can clarify ambiguous MCQs and highlight leading contenders for this years' essay titles.

Groups do present their own problems. Choose carefully who you are going to study with, to maximize your own chances of passing. It is best to work with people that you get on with and you know that you can work with collaboratively. The size of the group is also important. We recommend a group of three or four as ideal. Less than this is not much better than studying alone, whereas a larger group can become inefficient and the benefits diffused too widely between members. It is useful to set an agenda before each meeting to make maximum use of the limited time.

It is likely that academic activities in your area, such as case presentations or journal clubs, will provide material relevant to the exam. Attending these activities also gives you an opportunity to hear the opinions of senior colleagues, some of whom may well be examiners.

Timetable and recommended texts

When to start revision for the Part II MRCPsych is a matter for individual discretion. However, 12 weeks' preparation is an absolute minimum. It should be borne in mind that taking the Part II MRCPsych is an expensive process, and that the highest chance of success is at the first attempt. Thus it makes sense to put everything into that first attempt, and not put yourself forward as a candidate prematurely.

Many candidates find it useful to use one or more of the major textbooks as a guide to the topics to be worked through; alternatively the exam syllabus, which is available from the College, may be used in this way. As none of the textbooks available covers enough material, or is up to date enough, it is necessary to gain information from an array of other sources.

Early preparation should include reading the *British Journal of Psychiatry* editorials, which often highlight developing and fashionable issues. If the *British Journal of Psychiatry* is not available in your local hospital library, it is worth considering joining the Royal College of Psychiatrists as an inceptor, which includes a subscription to the *Journal*. You should also look at appropriate editorials and reviews in the *Psychiatric Bulletin*, the *Lancet*, the *British Medical Journal*, *Current Opinion in Psychiatry*; and *Advances in Psychiatric Treatment* from the last 2–3 years

Other reading should focus on the major textbooks: you will get an idea of which textbooks we feel are appropriate by noting our source references for the MCQs. We have generally stuck to books and references that are widely available. When choosing a standard revision text it is important to note how contemporaneous the latest edition is, as the whole field of neurosciences is rapidly advancing.

Throughout the period of exam revision it is essential to acquire and practice as many MCQs as are available to you. They give an indication of the breadth and depth of knowledge expected of you. The questions can be used to guide study and to take you into areas that are particularly well suited to examination by this method. Spicing up your reading by occasional forays into MCQs alleviates boredom and allows you to identify gaps and weaknesses in your knowledge base.

In the crucial last week of preparation, its probably best to go over your revision notes and model essays. It is also worth continuing with MCQs, as long as you recognize that your normal mood swings at success and failure will be exacerbated.

Exam technique

The much vexed question of exam technique usually leads to a plethora of advice for the already confused candidate.

MCQ technique has long been known to be a vital ingredient to overall success. However, techniques vary from the ultra-safe 'only answer those you are 100% certain about' to the scatter-gun 'answer everything' approach. Research (Harden *et al.* 1976, Fleming 1988) has shown that educated guessing, or 'backing your hunches', improves the total overall score in a negatively marked multiple true/false MCQ such as the MRCPsych. In fact, when candidates were instructed to answer absolutely all items in this sort of an exam, many more gained than lost marks. Also, it is worth remembering that we never learn false information, so it could be argued that answers that turn out to be false might be harder to mark confidently than true answers.

In the presentation of our questions we allow the reader to grade the certainty of their answer. This should encourage an answer to every item, with an outright guess presumably being assigned a 'low' certainty. By following this method the reader will be able to calculate for themselves how 'good' they are at guessing. By repeating this exercise throughout the book it should become possible to develop an individual threshold for 'backing your hunches' or knowing when to commit to your guesses. We believe this is crucial, not only for the final total mark, but also the self-confidence required in the heat of the exam.

The other advice commonly prescribed is to hunt for clues to the correct response within the wording of the original question. Table 1 was applied to a series of negatively-marked medical MCQs without using any medical knowledge, and yielded a positive mark of 9%.

The day of the exam

After all these months of preparation, leave nothing to chance. If the exam centre is some distance away, make sure that you know how to get there and that your travel arrangements give you plenty of time. The last thing you want is to arrive at the exam late and already under pressure, after sitting in a traffic jam or on a delayed train.

On the big day itself remember state-dependent learning; that is, if you normally work best after two cups of coffee, remember to drink two cups of coffee prior to the exam.

When first confronted by the actual paper, avoid the temptation to skim through the questions seeking the reassurance of an easy MCQ. Much better to work through the paper systematically. Remember your first response on deliberation is likely to be your best. It may be worth actually taking a piece of blank card into the

Table 1   Positive and negative key words and phrases (reproduced with permission from Slade and Dewey, 1983)

True responses	False responses
May	Always
May be	Necessarily
Can be	Is necessary
Can appear	Characteristically
Tend(s)	Typically
Contributes to	All
Is of benefit	First
Of value	Appropriate
Useful	Same as
Suggest(s)	The fact that
Is possible	Do(es) not
Encourages	Requires
Are (is) often	No value
Are (is) frequently	Are free from
Have (has) been	Is complete
Usually	Very useful
	Is important
	Essential

exam which can be used to cover any items or questions lower down the page. This will decrease your distraction from the item requiring scrutiny.

Budget your time appropriately, although most candidates finish easily within the allotted span.

The MCQ papers are at the end of the day after two other exacting papers. Unlike the essay and critical review papers, time is rarely a major problem in the MCQ so there is no necessity to race through each paper. Do not be disheartened if it seems initially that many of the questions are obscure, this is a common feeling, particularly in the basic science paper, and it is the same for everyone.

After answering the easy questions go through the paper again answering those you feel are above your 'certainty threshold' as previously determined when practising with this book. Avoid changing too many answers as often your first thoughts are correct. Once you have completed the paper, it is worth reviewing your responses just one time, to exclude any accidental mistakes. We caution against changing many of your responses.

Some candidates calculate the proportion of the paper they have answered, usually with a rough target in mind (which should be more than 50%!). This is fine but should be informed by the comments given above.

Good luck!

References

Fleming, P.R. (1988) The profitability of 'guessing' in multiple choice question papers. *Medical Education* 22, 509–513.

Harden, R., Brown, R.A. *et al.* (1976) Multiple choice questions: to guess or not to guess. *Medical Education.* 10, 27–31.

Slade, P.D. and Dewey, M.E. (1983) Role of grammatical clues in multiple choice questions: an empirical study. *Medical Teacher* 5(4), 146–148.

QBase* *Psychiatry on CD-ROM*

System requirements

- IBM-compatible PC with a minimum 80386 processor and 4Mb of RAM
- VGA monitor (or higher) set up to display at least 256 colours (N.B. The display setting of your computer must be set to display 'SMALL FONTS')
- CD-ROM drive
- Windows 3.1 or higher with Microsoft compatible mouse

Installation instructions

- The program will install the appropriate files on to your hard drive. It requires the QBase CD-ROM to be installed in the CD-ROM (usually D:) drive.
- **In order to run QBase the CD-ROM must be in the drive**.
- Print **readme.txt** and **helpfile.txt** on the CD-ROM for further instructions and user manual.

Windows 95/98

1 Insert the QBase CD-ROM into the CD-ROM **drive (usually D:)**
2 From the **Start Menu**, select the **Run** option
3 Type **D:\setup.exe** and press **Enter** or **Return**
4 **Follow the Full Installation option** and accept the default directory for installation of QBase. The installation program creates a folder called **QBaseOUP** containing the program icon and another called **Exams** into which you can save previous exam attempts.
5 To run QBase, double click the **QBaseOUP** icon in the QBase folder. From Windows Explorer double click the **QBaseOUP.exe** file in the QBase folder.

*QBase Interactive MCQ Examinations © 1996 E. Hammond/Greenwich Medical Media Ltd

Windows 3.1/Windows for Workgroups 3.11

1 Insert the QBase CD-ROM into the CD-ROM **drive (usually D:)**
2 From the **File Menu**, select the **Run** option
3 Type **D:\setup.exe** and press **Enter** or **Return**
4 Follow the instructions given by the installation program. Select the **Full Installation** option and accept the default directory for installation of QBase. The installation program creates a program window and directory called **QBaseOUP** containing the program icon. It also creates a directory called **Exams** into which you can save previous examination atttempts.
5 To run QBase, double click on the **QBaseOUP** icon in the QBaseOUP program window. From File Manager double click the **QBaseOUP.exe** file in the QBaseOUP directory.

Paper 1

Basic science

1.1

[Certainty]

Neurofibrillary tangles

	High	Med	Low
a Are formed within nerve cell bodies.	...	...	...
b Are particularly seen in Ammon's horn.	...	...	...
c Can be a part of normal ageing.	...	...	...
d Have amyloid in the paired helical filaments.	...	...	...
e Particularly characterize pre-senile Alzheimer's disease.	...	...	...

1.2

A computed tomography (CT) head scan

a Delivers the equivalent radiation of 100 chest X-rays.	...	...	...
b Lasts about 15 minutes.	...	...	...
c Is good at detecting white matter lesions.	...	...	...
d Is the investigation of choice for a suspected brain stem lesion.	...	...	...
e Needs reversed axial views for optimal viewing of the temporal lobes.	...	...	...

1.3

Cerebral tumours that present with psychiatric symptomatology are more likely to be

a Meningiomas than gliomas.	...	...	...
b Slow growing tumours.	...	...	...
c Benign than malignant.	...	...	...
d Infratentorial than supratentorial.	...	...	...
e Frontal lobe in site when associated with impairment of consciousness.	...	...	...

Paper 1: Answers

Basic science

1.1

a **True.** Particularly in the pyramidal cells of the hippocampus, where they are flame-shaped.

b **True.** Also found in the amygdala, neocortex, locus coeruleus, parahippocampal gyrus, and raphe nuclei.

c **True.** Apart from Alzheimer's disease, tangles are seen in Down's syndrome, dementia pugilistica, supranuclear palsy, and postencephalitic Parkinson's disease.

d **False.** Amyloid, which is formed from an aggregation of beta A4 protein deposits, characterizes senile plaques. Neurofibrillary tangles are composed of paired helical filaments, and may also accumulate around plaques.

e **False.** The histology of early and late onset Alzheimer's disease is much the same. The number and neocortical extent of plaques and tangles has been thought to reflect disease stage.

Lishman, W.A. (1998) *Organic psychiatry*, 3rd edn. Blackwell Science, Oxford, pp. 440–441.

Morgan, G. and Butler, S. (eds.) (1993) *Seminars in basic neurosciences*. Gaskell, London, pp. 198–201.

1.2

a **True.** The risk of ionizing radiation can be overlooked. The lens of the eye is particularly vulnerable, leading to cataracts. Pregnancy is not an absolute contraindication to a CT scan, however.

b **True.**

c **False.** Although not yet widely available, magnetic resonance imaging (MRI) is superseding CT as a first choice imaging modality. Exceptions to this are bony and calcified lesions, and fresh haemorrhages.

d **False.** MRI is better for posterior fossa and brain stem imaging. MRI images are not degraded by bony artefact.

e **True.** If MRI is unavailable, these views can be specifically requested.

Morgan, G. and Butler, S. (eds.) (1993) *Seminars in Basic Neurosciences*. Gaskell, London, pp. 302–314.

1.3

a **False.** Gliomas more than meningiomas

b **False.** Rapidly growing tumours.

c **False.** Probably related to the greater incidence of raised intracranial pressure.

d **False.** Supratentorial more than infratentorial

e **True.**

Lishman, W.A. (1998). *Organic psychiatry*, 3rd edn. Blackwell Science, Oxford, pp. 220–221.

Questions

1.4

	[Certainty]		
Maternally deprived infant rhesus monkeys	High	Med	Low
a Are outwardly aggressive (i.e. hiss and spit) at strangers which pass by their cage.	...	...	...
b Are sexually competent.	...	...	...
c Have poor maternal skills.	...	...	...
d Incorrectly interpret the emotions of their fellow monkeys.	...	...	...
e Develop neuronal morphological change.	...	...	...

1.5

According to Parson's theory of the 'sick role', the individual sufferer

	High	Med	Low
a Must want to get well as soon as possible.	...	...	...
b Should seek professional medical advice and cooperate with the doctor.	...	...	...
c Is allowed (and may be expected) to shed some normal activities and responsibilities (e.g. employment and household tasks).	...	...	...
d Is regarded as being in need of care and unable to get better by his or her decision and will.	...	...	...
e May adopt the role as a permanent state if they have a chronic illness.	...	...	...

1.6

The 'Black' report

	High	Med	Low
a Was commissioned to examine health in different ethnic groups.	...	...	...
b Reported higher mortality rates in lower socio-economic classes.	...	...	...
c Found higher sickness rates in skilled and professional workers.	...	...	...
d Concluded that the NHS provided equal access for all social classes to healthcare.	...	...	...
e Was commissioned by a Labour government and published during a Conservative one.	...	...	...

Answers

1.4

   a **False.** Normal monkeys hiss and spit. Maternally deprived monkeys retreat to the back of their cage and tend to harm themselves (bite their limbs, etc.).

   b **False.** Males show no interest in females and fail to complete copulation.

   c **True.** Mothers are intolerant of their offspring and do not allow intimacy.

   d **True.** This was demonstrated in task learning by operant conditioning involving two monkeys working co-operatively.

   e **True.**

Weller, M. and Eysenck, M. (1991) *The scientific basis of psychiatry*, 2nd edn. Saunders, Phildelphia, pp. 446–447.

1.5

   a **True.**

   b **True.**

   c **True.**

   d **True.**

   e **False.** Parsons viewed the sick role as temporary. Those with chronic illness are not expected to occupy the sick role permanently, but at times of exacerbations of illness.

Tantum, D. and Birchwood, M. (eds.) (1994) *Seminars in psychology and the social sciences*. Gaskell, London, pp. 319–320.

1.6

   a **False.** It was to look at inequality in health between different socio-economic groups.

   b **True.**

   c **False.** Higher sickness rates were in unskilled and semi-skilled groups.

   d **False.** It made the opposite conclusion.

   e **True.**

Kendell, R.E. and Zealley, A.K. (eds.) (1993) *Companion to psychiatric studies*, 5th edn. Churchill Livingstone, Edinburgh, p. 13.

Department. of Health and Social Security (1980) *Inequalities in health: Report of a research working group*. HMSO, London.

Questions
1.7

[Certainty]

In a randomized clinical trial

	High	Med	Low
a All subjects have the same probability of receiving each of the different forms of treatment.	...	...	...
b The allocation of subjects is not influenced by investigator bias.	...	...	...
c No one knows the treatment allocation in a double blind trial.	...	...	...
d The effects of variables other than the treatment under study are randomly distributed between comparison groups.	...	...	...
e The randomization code should be held distant from the site of investigation.	...	...	...

1.8

The following statements regarding disease prevalence and incidence are correct.

	High	Med	Low
a The point prevalence is the proportion of a defined population that has a disease during a given time interval.	...	...	...
b The birth defect rate is the proportion of aborted fetuses that have chromosomal abnormalities.	...	...	...
c Incidence is calculated by dividing the number of new cases over the given time period by the total population at risk.	...	...	...
d Relative risk refers to the ratio of the incidence of a disease in people exposed to the risk factor to the incidence of a disease in people not exposed to the same risk factor.	...	...	...
e The attributable risk is the same as the odds ratio.	...	...	...

1.9

Population studies of the elderly have found:

	High	Med	Low
a A prevalence of dementia of 1% in those under 65 years old.	...	...	...
b A prevalence of dementia of greater than 30% in those aged over 90 years old.	...	...	...
c That the risk of developing dementia increases linearly with increasing age.	...	...	...
d The prevalence of dementia doubles approximately every 5 years.	...	...	...
e Vascular risk factors to be important in the onset of Alzheimer's disease.	...	...	...

Answers
1.7

   a **True.** The randomized double-blind controlled clinical trial is now held to be the gold standard of clinical trials, and the cornerstone of evidence-based medicine.

   b **True.** As opposed to using volunteer controls or historical controls.

   c **False.** No one participating directly in the study should have access to the allocation code, but it must exist!

   d **True.** These variables may well be unknown, but in a large study can rightly be assumed to be evenly distributed across comparison groups.

   e **True.** To avoid corrupt investigators influencing the study by cracking the code.

Puri, B. and Hall, A.D. (1998) *Revision notes in psychiatry* 6. Arnold, London, p. 61.

1.8

   a **False.** The point prevalence is the proportion of a defined population that has a disease at a given point in time.

   b **False.** The birth defect rate is the proportion of live births that has a given disease.

   c **True.**

   d **True.**

   e **False.** The attributable risk is also known as the risk difference or absolute excess risk. The odds ratio is a measure of relative risk in retrospective epidemiological samples.

Puri, B. and Tyrer, P. (1992) *Sciences basic to psychiatry*. Churchill Livingstone, Edinburgh, pp. 269–271.

1.9

   a **True.** The prevalence is the number of people of a defined population that have a disease at a given point in time, divided by the total number of people at risk.

   b **True.**

   c **False.** The increase is exponential.

   d **True.**

   e **True.**

Holmes, C. and Howard, R. (eds.) (1997) *Advances in old age psychiatry*. Wrightson Biomedical, Stroud, pp. 3–17.

Questions
1.10

	[Certainty]		
The chi-squared (χ^2) test:	High	Med	Low

a Is a non-parametric test.

b Can be used to detect the differences between percentages.

c Is used to test the null hypothesis.

d Can be a '2 $\times$ 2' table.

e Requires a Yates correction if numbers are large.

1.11

Restriction fragment length polymorphisms (RFLPs)

a Can be used as genetic markers.

b Can be produced by Southern blotting.

c Are generally inherited in a simple Mendelian fashion.

d Are usually multi-allelic.

e Allow mutations to be easily characterized.

1.12

The reticular formation is

a Involved in the regulation of aggression.

b Related neurochemically to the raphe nuclei.

c Known to cause arousal from sleep by blocking the rhythmical synchronous neuronal discharging of the cortex, via the thalamus.

d Situated in the brain stem.

e Known to have projections to nearly half of the cortex.

Answers
1.10

a **True.** That is, the data are not normally distributed.
b **False.** Only on actual numbers of occurrences.
c **True.** The null hypothesis states that there are no differences between the populations being studied.
d **True.** Also known as a 'fourfold' table.
e **False.** The Yates continuity correction should be used if the total of the cells is less than 100 or any cell has a value of less than 10.

Swinscow, T.D.V. (1983) *Statistics at square one.* BMJ Publications. London, pp. 43–53.

1.11

a **True.** Variations in the size of specific restriction fragments of DNA labelled by a given probe after Southern blotting are termed restriction fragment length polymorphisms (RFLPs) . They are generally inherited in a simple Mendelian fashion and so can be used as genetic markers.
b **True.** Southern blotting is named after its inventor E M Southern. Genomic DNA is cut with a restriction enzyme which produces a large number of different sized DNA fragments. These can be separated by size by gel electrophoresis.
c **True.** The different alleles of the genetic markers can be distinguished and their inheritance followed through families or studied in populations.
d **False.** The majority of RFLPs arise from single base substitutions and are bi-allelic.
e **False.** Gross abnormalities can be detected via Southern blotting, and point mutations may be seen by DNA sequencing. PCR (polymerase chain reaction) type techniques allow identification of known mutations.

McGuffin, P., Owen, M.J., O'Donovan, M.C., Thapar, A. and Gottesman, I.I. (1994) *Seminars in psychiatric genetics.* Gaskell, London, pp. 18–22.

1.12

a **False.** Studies suggest that the amygdala has an excitatory effect on aggression. The reticular formation is principally concerned with arousal.
b **True.** The raphe nuclei are situated in the midline of the pons and medulla, and primarily their axons operate using 5-HT. Lesions of the raphe nuclei and 5-HT depleting drugs lead to insomnia.
c **True.** This repetitive synchronous discharge prevents cortical neurones from participating in the processing of cognitive and perceptual information, leading to one being unconscious during sleep.
d **True.** It is a core of grey matter surrounding the aqueduct of Silvius.
e **False.** There are connections with all of the cortex.

Morgan, G. and Butler, S. (eds.) (1993) *Seminars in basic neurosciences.* Gaskell, London, pp. 39–40.

Questions

1.13

[Certainty]

The following neuroanatomical statements are true.   High   Med   Low

  a Giant cells of Betz are located in the prefrontal area.   ...   .

  b The auditory association cortex is involved in
     interpretation of symbolic sound patterns.   ...   .

  c Association fibres are only intra-hemispheric.   ...   .

  d Histologically, the hippocampus is a six-layered
     structure.   ...   .

  e The IIIrd cranial nerve includes sympathetic fibres.   ...   .

1.14

The following regions of the hypothalamus are correctly paired
with their presumed function:

  a Lateral zone and satiety.   ...   .

  b Medial zone and the 'hunger centre'.   ...   .

  c Periventricular area and sexual behaviour.   ...   .

  d Medial forebrain bundle (MFB) and temperature
     regulation.   ...   .

  e Anterior hypothalamus and the 'pleasure centre'.   ...   .

1.15

The following are involved in the γ-aminobutyrate (GABA)
shunt

  a Glutamate.   ...   .

  b Pyridoxal phosphate.   ...   .

  c 6-Phosphogluconate.   ...   .

  d Succinate.   ...   .

  e Tyrosine hydroxylase.   ...   .

Answers
1.13

   a **True.** They are found in the primary motor cortex.

   b **True.** It is the secondary auditory area and is adjacent to the primary auditory area.

   c **True.** As compared with commissural fibres.

   d **False.** Three-layered, molecular (superficial), pyramidal and polymorphic.

   e **False.** Parasympathetic fibres are present in cranial nerves 2, 3, 7, 9 and 10.

Puri, B. and Tyrer, P. (1992) Sciences basic to psychiatry. Churchill Livingstone, Edinburgh, pp. 11–20.

1.14

   a **False.** The satiety centre is thought to be in the medial zone.

   b **False.** The hunger centre is thought to be in the lateral zone.

   c **True.**

   d **False.** The MFB is thought to be associated with pleasure.

   e **False.** The anterior hypothalamus is involved with temperature regulation.

Puri, B. and Tyrer, P. (1992) *Sciences basic to psychiatry*. Churchill Livingstone, Edinburgh, pp. 40–43.

1.15

   a **True.**

   b **True.** Pyridoxal phosphate is the vitamin B_6 derived cofactor for glutamic acid decarboxylase.

   c **False.** 6-Phosphogluconate is involved in the pentose phosphate pathway.

   d **True.**

   e **False.** Tyrosine hydroxylase is involved in the biosynthetic pathway of the catecholamines.

Note: Glutamate —(1)→ GABA —(2)→ succinate semialdehyde —(3)→ succinate

(1) Glutamic acid decarboxylase

(2) GABA-glutamate transaminase

(3) Succinate semialdehyde dehydrogenase

Puri, B. and Tyrer, P. (1992) *Sciences basic to psychiatry*. Churchill Livingstone, Edinburgh, pp. 90–91.

Questions

1.16

The following are a consequence of a plasma lithium level of over 2 mmol l⁻¹	High	Med	Low
a Oliguria.	...	...	...
b Fine tremor.	...	...	...
c Oedema.	...	...	...
d Syncope.	...	...	...
e Acute renal failure.	...	...	...

1.17

With regard to antidepressant medication

a Fluoxetine may be used in renal failure.	...	...	...
b Fluvoxamine, paroxetine, and sertraline have similar half lives.	...	...	...
c Trazodone is an example of an azaspirodecanedione.	...	...	...
d Mianserin possesses no cardiotoxic effects.	...	...	...
e Theophylline toxicity may result from co-administration of a serotonin re-uptake inhibitor.	...	...	...

1.18

Serotonin or 5-hydroxytryptamine (5HT)

a Is a monoamine neurotransmitter.	...	...	...
b Is hydroxylated tryptophan.	...	...	...
c Can be depleted in the brain by adding extra alanine to the diet.	...	...	...
d Has been linked to type 1 alcoholism.	...	...	...
e Is degraded via 5-hydroxyindoleacetic acid.	...	...	...

Answers
1.16

a **True.** Polyuria (and polydipsia) are well recognized side-effects of therapeutic lithium levels, rather than intoxication.

b **False.** Fine tremor is a side-effect, whereas a coarse tremor occurs in intoxication. However, plasma levels of >2 mmol l^{-1} are dangerous, and hyperreflexia, fits, and even coma and death can occur.

c **False.** Again, a side-effect.

d **True.** Syncope and circulatory collapse can lead to coma, hence urgent medical attention is required.

e **False.** Although lithium is nephrotoxic, this is more usual in the chronic scenario. Concomitant thiazide or loop diuretic therapy should be avoided, as these reduce lithium excretion.

Puri, B. (1995) *Saunders' pocket essentials of psychiatry.* Saunders, Philadelphia, p. 97.

1.17

a **False.** There may be an accumulation of the drug and its metabolites.

b **True.** Approximately 24 hours. The half life of fluoxetine is 48–72 hours.

c **False.** A triazolopyridine.

d **True.** Mianserin has been associated with leucopenia, agranulocytosis, and aplastic anaemia. A full blood count is recommended every 4 weeks for the first 3 months and regularly thereafter.

e **True.** Inhibits metabolism by oxidative microsomsal liver enzymes..

British National Formulary, Sections 4.3.1, 4.3.3, appendices 1 and 3 .

Gelder, M., Gath, D., Mayou, R., and Cowen, P. (eds.) (1996) *The Oxford textbook of psychiatry*, 3rd edn. Oxford University Press, Oxford, pp. 566, 574.

1.18

a **True.** Along with dopamine and noradrenaline. 5-HT neurones originate in several brainstem nuclei, particularly the dorsal and median raphe.

b **False.** The dietary amino acid L-tryptophan is first converted to 5-hydroxytryptophan by tryptophan hydroxylase, and then 5-HT is produced via 5-HTP decarboxylase. Neither of these enzymes is saturated, so the availability of L-tryptophan is rate-limiting.

c **True.** Adding a neutral amino acid such as alanine, which competes for the same transport processes, blocks the entry of L-tryptophan into the brain. Conversely, lowering plasma concentrations of these neutral amino acids augments L-tryptophan entry into the CNS.

d **False.** A number of studies (particularly from Finland) have linked the 'low serotonin syndrome' with Cloninger's type 2 alcoholism (young alcoholic males prone to antisocial and impulsive behaviour).

e **True.** 5-hydroxyindoleacetic acid (5HIAA) is transported out of the brain via the blood or CSF. 5HIAA is easier to measure in the CSF than 5HT, and low CSF levels of 5HIAA have been linked to suicide and impulsivity.

Morgan, G. and Butler, S. (eds.) (1993) *Seminars in basic neurosciences.* Gaskell, London, pp. 102–107.

Questions

1.19

	[Certainty]		
In the electroencephalogram (EEG)	High	Med	Low
a Beta activity is at a frequency of 8–12 Hz.	...	...	...
b Alpha activity is found mainly in the frontal areas.	...	...	...
c Benzodiazepines will reduce β activity.	...	...	...
d μ activity occurs maximally over the precentral gyrus.	...	...	...
e Chlorpromazine will increase delta activity.	...	...	...

1.20

In the narcolepsy/cataplexy syndrome

	High	Med	Low
a Routine electroencephalography (EEG) shows no abnormality in narcolepsy.	...	...	...
b Narcolepsy has characteristic findings on polysomnography.	...	...	...
c Pharmacological intervention is unhelpful for cataplexy.	...	...	...
d Hypnogogic hallucinations are required to make the diagnosis of narcolepsy.	...	...	...
e Strong emotion may bring on narcolepsy attacks.	...	...	...

1.21

The following are examples of G-protein coupled receptors:

	High	Med	Low
a $5HT_2$ receptors.	...	...	...
b Adrenergic receptors.	...	...	...
c Cholinergic muscarinic receptors.	...	...	...
d GABA type A receptors.	...	...	...
e Glycine receptors.	...	...	...

1.22

In the field of human perception research

	High	Med	Low
a The 'just noticeable difference' divided by stimulus intensity is the Weber fraction.	...	...	...
b Weber's fractions are largest for the sense of hearing.	...	...	...
c Weber's law states that the relationship between a standard stimulus and a 'just noticeable difference' in that stimulus produces a constant ratio.	...	...	...
d Fechner's law states that the strength of a sensation grows as the square of the stimulus intensity.	...	...	...
e Signal detection theory states that perception does not depend only on stimulus intensity.	...	...	...

Answers
1.19

a **False.** Beta activity is at a frequency greater than or equal to 13 Hz.

b **False.** Alpha activity is found mainly in the occipital areas It is also known as 'Berger' rhythm.

c **False.** Benzodiazepines will increase beta activity thereby reducing the tendency to seizures.

d **True.** The motor cortex. It is abolished by movements in the contralateral limb.

e **True.** Causing a slowing of the EEG, therefore reducing the seizure threshold.

Puri, B. and Tyrer, P. (1992) *Sciences basic to psychiatry*. Churchill Livingstone, Edinburgh, pp. 63–65.

1.20

a **True.**

b **True.** There is a direct entry into rapid eye movement (REM) sleep.

c **False.** The frequency of attacks may be helped by tricyclic antidepressants.

d **False.** They are present in 30% of sufferers.

e **False.** Strong emotion may precipitate cataplexy (sudden, temporary muscle paralysis) but not narcolepsy.

Lishman, W.A. (1998) *Organic psychiatry*, 3rd edn. Blackwell Science, Oxford, pp. 721–727.

1.21

a **True.** G-proteins are cellular proteins that link cell surface receptors to various enzymes and ion channels. Note $5HT_{1A, B, C}$ and $5HT_3$ are ligand gated ion channel receptors.

b **True.**

c **True.** Nicotinic receptors are ligand gated ion channel receptors.

d **False.** GABA type A is a ligand-gated ionic channel receptor. GABA type B is G-protein coupled.

e **False.** Glycine is a ligand-gated ionic channel receptor .

Kendell, R.E. and Zealley, A.K. (eds.) (1993) *Companion to psychiatric studies*, 5th edn. Churchill Livingstone, Edinburgh, pp. 113–115.

1.22

a **True.**

b **False.** Smell, i.e. a larger change in stimulus is necessary to detect a difference.

c **True.**

d **False.** The strength of a sensation grows as the logarithm of the stimulus intensity.

e **True.** Other factors are important such as motivation and previous experiences.

Puri, B. and Tyrer, P. (1992) *Sciences basic to psychiatry*. Churchill Livingstone, Edinburgh, pp. 278–279.

Questions
1.23

	[Certainty]		
The following statements concerning memory are true:	High	Med	Low
a Short-term memory (STM) has an unlimited capacity.	...	...	...
b Items must enter short-term memory first before being able to enter long-term memory.	...	...	...
c With long-term memory, recall is superior to recognition.	...	...	...
d Interference of previously learnt information is the most important factor which can impair retrieval of memory.	...	...	...
e 'Working memory' is thought to be a part of long-term memory.	...	...	...

1.24

Studies of human attachment have shown the following:			
a Parental temperament is the best predictor of the nature of the attachment between child and parent.	...	...	...
b The majority of children assessed were shown to be securely attached at 14 months old.	...	...	...
c Those 14 month old children who were deemed 'avoidant' in attachment type typically ignored the mother, and avoided interaction with her.	...	...	...
d Children found to be 'avoidant' during the strange situation were at much higher risk of later schizophrenia.	...	...	...
e In the home environment, categorical differences in the mothers were observed.	...	...	...

1.25

In social psychology			
a The social exchange theory refers to satisfaction in interpersonal relationships.	...	...	...
b Rusbult's investment model states that a relationship will be stronger the more protected time a couple have together.	...	...	...
c Women with more attractive partners have been found to be less neurotic than women with less attractive partners.	...	...	...
d Married couples tend to be similar in terms of physical attractiveness.	...	...	...
e Interdependence theory postulates that people will be more attracted to another and will be more satisfied with the relationship if the outcome is more positive than expected.	...	...	...

Answers

1.23

a **False.** STM has a limited storage capacity (5–9 items).

b **False.** This is not necessarily the case. Various experiments have shown that subjects with poor STM (amnesic syndrome) can assimilate information into LTM.

c **False.** Recognition is superior to recall.

d **True.**

e **False.** Thought to be part of STM.

Kendell, R.E. and Zealley, A.K. (eds.) (1993) *Companion to psychiatric studies*, 5th edn. Churchill Livingstone, Edinburgh, pp. 31–32.

1.24

a **False.** This statement is true, but does not relate to the 'strange situation' test.

b **True.** The Ainsworth 'strange situation' test is an influential but criticized method of assessing attachment. It measures the child's behaviour at separation from, and reunion with the caregiver. 66% of children were described as 'securely attached', which means they were distressed and not exploratory at maternal separation, but showed pleasure and proximity-seeking behaviour on reunion with mother.

c **True.** 20% of those children assessed in the strange environment.

d **False.** No follow-up studies from the 'strange situation' are available. However, the description of the mothers of those children 'ambivalent' in the strange situation is reminiscent of the 'double bind' theory, i.e. inconsistent and insensitive mothering.

e **True.** The value of these judgements is dubious.

Tantum, D. and Birchwood, M. (eds.) (1994) *Seminars in psychology and the social sciences*. Gaskell, London, pp. 159–161.

1.25

a **True.** People have preference for relationships that appear to offer an optimum cost : benefit ratio.

b **False.** Rusbult proposed that the commitment to a relationship will be stronger the better the outcome, the fewer the alternatives and the greater the investment.

c **True.**

d **True.**

e **True.**

Tantum, D. and Birchwood, M. (eds.) (1994) *Seminars in psychology and the social sciences*. Gaskell, London, pp. 168–178.

Questions

Clinical

1.26
[Certainty]

The following are common sequelae of a severe head injury with   High   Med   Low
a post-traumatic amnesia of greater than 24 hours:

  a Delirium.

  b Personality change.

  c Depression.

  d Schizophrenia-like syndrome.

  e Lasting cognitive impairment.

1.27

Significant cognitive decline in people infected with the human
immunodeficiency virus (HIV)

  a Usually occurs only with significant immunosuppression.

  b Occurs early in the course of infection.

  c Has been shown to be helped by the antiretroviral drug
      AZT.

  d Can be due to HIV encephalitis.

  e Occurs in less than 10% of people with AIDS.

1.28

A temporal lobe focus is suggested by an aura consisting of

  a Lip-smacking.

  b Forced thinking.

  c Lilliputian hallucinations.

  d Tinnitus.

  e Loss of consciousness.

Answers

Clinical

1.26

a **True.** An impairment of consciousness, accompanied by changes in affect, and disturbances in perception and the sleep–wake cycle.

b **True.** Particularly after frontal lobe damage. Irritability, lack of drive, and poor impulse control may make management difficult and increase the burden on relatives.

c **True.** Persistent changes in affect are said to occur in up to a quarter of patients. Note that suicide risk is also increased after head injury.

d **False.** The rate of schizophrenia-like syndrome is above that expected but is not common.

e **True.** After a closed injury the impairment is usually global. Penetrating injuries may be associated with more focal cognitive deficits, dependent upon location of injury.

Gelder, M., Gath, D., Mayou, R., and Cowen, P. (eds.) (1996) *The Oxford textbook of psychiatry*, 3rd edn. Oxford University Press, Oxford, pp. 326–328.

1.27

a **True.**

b **False.** It tends to occur later in the clinical course.

c **True.**

d **True.**

e **False.** The figure is closer to one third.

King, M. (1993) *AIDS, HIV, and mental health*. Cambridge University Press, Cambridge, pp. 57–72.

1.28

a **True.**

b **True.**

c **True.**

d **True.**

e **False.**

Note: Temporal lobe auras are complex and varied. They may or may not lead onto a motor convulsion. There is usually subtle clouding of consciousness, rather than loss. Sometimes post-ictal automatisms are seen.

A history of birth injury or infantile febrile convulsions may be obtained. Attacks show increased incidence through adolescence to early adult life.

Seizure-induced anoxia may further damage the hippocampus, and at surgery mesial sclerosis is often found. Medication-resistant cases may be surgically remediable.

Mace, C. (1993) Epilepsy and schizophrenia. *British Journal of Psychiatry* 163, 439–446.

Questions

1.29

	[Certainty]		
In the elderly	High	Med	Low
a The suicide rate is similar in males and females.	...	...	...
b Parasuicide is rare and has an almost equal sex incidence.	...	...	...
c 'Open space phobia' is well recognized.	...	...	...
d Syllogomania is also known as senile squalor syndrome.	...	...	...
e ECT is contraindicated in moderate dementia.	...	...	...

1.30

The drug 'Ecstasy'

a Commonly causes hallucinations.	...	...	...
b Is 3,4-methylenedioxy-methamphetamine.	...	...	...
c Is a controlled drug in the UK.	...	...	...
d Has an effect which lasts for several hours.	...	...	...
e Causes neuronal serotonin depletion in animal studies.	...	...	...

1.31

Caffeine

a Is the most widely used psychoactive drug in the world.	...	...	...
b Withdrawal symptoms include impaired psychomotor performance.	...	...	...
c Withdrawal starts at 1–2 hours post ingestion.	...	...	...
d Withdrawal symptoms are found commonly amongst heavy caffeine users.	...	...	...
e Intake in excess, is associated with problems in rehabilitating patients with chronic schizophrenia.	...	...	...

1.32

The following are true:

a The outcome of schizoaffective disorder has been found to be worse than that of schizophrenia or affective disorder.	...	...	...
b The incidence of affective illness is higher than schizophrenia in relatives of those with schizoaffective disorder.	...	...	...
c Paranoid illnesses occur more frequently than in the general population in those with poor auditory or visual acuity.	...	...	...
d Premorbid personality disorder is frequent in those developing a paranoid psychotic illness in old age.	...	...	...
e Schizophrenia is a common primary diagnosis in those suffering from erotomania.	...	...	...

Answers
1.29

a **False.** The male suicide rate is twice that of females and continues to increase with advancing age
b **True.**
c **True.** As described by Marks. Lack of available physical supports leads to anxiety. Usually have little confidence in their mobility but few background neurotic traits.
d **False.** This is compulsive collecting. The related Diogenes syndrome is senile squalor.
e **False.** Provided there is no space-occupying lesion.

Kendell, R.E. and Zealley, A.K. (eds.) (1993) *Companion to psychiatric studies,* 5th edn. Churchill Livingstone, Edinburgh, pp. 733–737.

1.30

a **False.** This is not a common effect.
b **True.**
c **True.** As an amphetamine-like drug.
d **True.**
e **True.** And possibly neuronal death.

Ghodse, A. H. and Kreek, M. J. (1997) A rave against ecstasy. *Current Opinion In Psychiatry* 10, 191–193.

1.31

a **True.**
b **True.**
c **False.** Starts at 12–24 hours and peaks at 1–2 days and normally lasts up to 1 week.
d **True.** Up to 100% of users.
e **True.** Withdrawal effects can mimic psychiatric symptoms.

Chick, J. and Cantwell, R. (eds.) (1994) *Seminars in alcohol and drug misuse.* Gaskell, London, pp. 72–73.

1.32

a **False.** Between the two.
b **True.**
c **True.** Especially in the elderly and in increased social isolation.
d **True.** A high proportion are unmarried, divorced, or widowed and many have lifelong abnormal personality traits.
e **True.**

Maj, M. & Perris, C. (1990) Patterns of course in patients with cross-sectional diagnosis of schizoaffective disorder. *Journal of Affective Disorders* 20 (2), 71–77.

Kendell, R.E. and Zealley, A.K. (eds.) (1993) *Companion to psychiatric studies,* 5th edn. Churchill Livingstone, Edinburgh, pp. 461–468.

Questions

1.33

	[Certainty]		
Bouffée délirante	High	Med	Low
a Is a transcultural syndrome.	...	...	...
b Rarely relapses.	...	...	...
c Usually has an insidious onset.	...	...	...
d Is recognized in ICD 10.	...	...	...
e Is characterized by a varying emotional state.	...	...	...

1.34

In postnatal psychiatric illness

a The overall suicide rate for women in their postnatal year is markedly increased.	...	...	...
b The severity of the 'baby blues' is associated with changes in oestrogen levels post partum.	...	...	...
c Premenstrual syndrome is more common in women who subsequently develop 'blues'	...	...	...
d Thyroid antibodies protect women against postnatal depression.	...	...	...
e Women developing postnatal depression have double the number of life-events in the preceding year.	...	...	...

1.35

In depressive disorder

a Depressed mood is required for a diagnosis of depressive disorder according to ICD 10.	...	...	...
b The risk of suicide is significantly greater in bipolar depression compared to unipolar depression.	...	...	...
c Depressive delusions predict a good response to ECT.	...	...	...
d Recurrence is more likely in females than males.	...	...	...
e 25% of patients with unipolar depression have a recurrence within 10 years of their first episode.	...	...	...

1.36

In transient global amnesia

a Attacks usually diminish after a few hours.	...	...	...
b Younger females are commonly affected.	...	...	...
c Confabulation is characteristic.	...	...	...
d Consciousness is clouded.	...	...	...
e Anxiety is commonly seen.	...	...	...

Answers
1.33

a **False.** Although originally described in France (literally 'a puff of madness'), there are other regional equivalents.

b **False.** It is thought to be a condition with a good prognosis, which is prone to relapse.

c **False.** Acute (<2 weeks) or abrupt (<48 hours) onset is defining, particularly after an associated stress within the same time-frame.

d **True.** Subsumed under 'acute polymorphic psychotic disorder' (F 23).

e **True.** As well as rapidly fluctuating psychotic phenomena.

World Health Organization (1992) *Tenth Revision of the International Classification of Disease (ICD 10)*. WHO, Geneva, pp. 101–102.

1.34

a **False.** It is significantly decreased.

b **False.** It is associated with the change in progesterone levels.

c **True.**

d **False.** Post natal depression occurs more often in women with thyroid antibodies.

e **True.**

Pritchard, D. B. and Harris, B. (1996) Aspects of perinatal psychiatric illness. *British Journal of Psychiatry* 169, 555–562.

1.35

a **False.**

b **False.** There is no conclusive evidence for this. Between 11% and 17% of persons with a severe depressive illness commit suicide.

c **True.** This was shown in the Northwick Park ECT trial.

d **True.**

e **False.** The figure is closer to 75%, supporting the view that depressive disorder does not have as a good prognosis as was once considered.

Gelder, M., Gath, D., Mayou, R., and Cowen, P. (eds.) (1996) *The Oxford textbook of psychiatry*, 3rd edn. Oxford University Press, Oxford, pp. 208–231.

1.36

a **True.** A vascular aetiology is postulated.

b **False.** Older males are commonly affected.

c **False.** Confabulation is rare.

d **False.** Consciousness is preserved.

e **True.** This is described as 'anxious bewilderment with repeated stereotyped questioning of onlookers'.

Lishman, W.A. (1998) *Organic psychiatry*, 3rd edn. Blackwell Science, Oxford, p. 413.

Questions

1.37

Regarding neurotic disorders

	[Certainty]		
	High	Med	Low
a In hypochondriacal disorder, the gastrointestinal system is most commonly involved.	...	...	...
b In somatization disorder, there is a preoccupation with the fear of having a specific illness.	...	...	...
c The sex ratio is equal in hypochondriasis.	...	...	...
d Sexual difficulties are almost universal in somatization disorder.	...	...	...
e Conversion disorders usually involve the cardiovascular system.	...	...	...

1.38

The following statements are true:

a The Epidemiological Catchment Area (ECA) study showed most neurotic disorders to have a peak occurrence in the 25–44 year age group.	...	...	...
b The onset of neurotic illnesses is related to an increase in total number of life events in the preceding 3 months.	...	...	...
c Sodium lactate has been used to ameliorate the symptoms of panic.	...	...	...
d Positron emission tomography (PET) has shown abnormal glucose metabolism in orbital frontal cortex and left caudate in subjects with obsessive–compulsive disorder compared to controls.	...	...	...
e Psychogenic amnesia is characterized by intact personal memories.	...	...	...

1.39

In structural family therapy

a The theory behind the therapy is associated with the work of Deschamps.	...	...	...
b The therapist observes the family and makes comments only at discrete intervals.	...	...	...
c A good family structure should have a clear hierarchy.	...	...	...
d There should be clear boundaries between sub-systems.	...	...	...
e Triangulation is helpful in facilitating communication within the family.	...	...	...

Answers

1.37

   a **False.** Musculoskeletal.

   b **False.** This is hypochondriacal disorder.

   c **True.**

   d **True.** Also menstrual problems.

   e **False.** Conversion disorders almost always involve the neurological system.

Gelder, M., Gath, D., Mayou, R., and Cowen, P. (eds.) (1996) *The Oxford textbook of psychiatry*, 3rd edn. Oxford University Press, Oxford, pp. 352–354.

1.38

   a **True.** The ECA was large collaborative study investigating the incidence and prevalence of various psychiatric diagnoses in America.

   b **True.**

   c **False.** Sodium lactate will induce symptoms of panic.

   d **True.**

   e **False.** Psychogenic amnesia is characterized by disturbed personal memories.

Kendell, R.E. and Zealley, A.K. (eds.) (1993) *Companion to psychiatric studies,* 5th edn. Churchill Livingstone, Edinburgh, pp. 485–514.

1.39

   a **False.** Minuchin.

   b **False.** The therapist is firmly in control of proceedings and is very active.

   c **True.** One of the central tenets of this type of therapy.

   d **True.**

   e **False.** This is a pathological process within families which can hinder effective communication.

Black, D. and Cottrell, D. (eds.) (1993) *Seminars in child and adolescent psychiatry.* Gaskell, London, pp. 198–200

Questions
1.40   [Certainty]

Features of Gilles de la Tourette's syndrome include	High	Med	Low
a Tremor.	...	...	...
b Echopraxia.	...	...	...
c A male preponderance.	...	...	...
d Coprophagia.	...	...	...
e An association with obsessive–compulsive disorder.	...	...	...

1.41

Fragile X syndrome

	High	Med	Low
a Is inherited as an X-linked recessive condition.	...	...	...
b Affects approximately 1 in 1000 females.	...	...	...
c Is characterized by CGG trinucleotide repeats.	...	...	...
d 1 in 5 males affected by the mutation are phenotypically and intellectually unaffected.	...	...	...
e Can present clinically with behaviour similar to attention deficit disorder.	...	...	...

1.42

Neuroleptic malignant syndrome is associated with

	High	Med	Low
a Low serum creatine phosphokinase.	...	...	...
b High serum iron.	...	...	...
c Lowered level of consciousness.	...	...	...
d A few specific antipsychotics.	...	...	...
e Breathing difficulty.	...	...	...

Answers
1.40

   a **False.** Although it may be associated with some of the treatments, e.g. antipsychotics.
   b **True.**
   c **True.**
   d **False.** Less than a third of clinic cases display coprolalia, echolalia, or echopraxia. Coprophagia means eating faeces.
   e **True.** Pedigree studies demonstrate an unusually high prevalence of OCD and Tourette's in families of affected probands. Neuroimaging work has suggested involvement of the frontal lobes, striatum, and caudate nucleii in both conditions.

Note: Multiple motor and vocal tics begin before the age of 18, usually at around 7 years old. There may be more complex stereotyped movements, like jumping. Associated features include attention deficit hyperactivity disorder, and emotional and social disturbances. Haloperidol is a long established treatment, which seems to help a proportion of patients.

Robertson, M.M. (1994) Annotation: Gilles de la Tourette's syndrome—an update. *Journal of Child Psychology and Psychiatry* 35(4), 597–611.

1.41

   a **False.** Is inherited as an atypical X-linked dominant condition.
   b **False.** It affects approximately 1 in 2000 females. Approximately 1 in 700 females is a carrier.
   c **True.** In the normal population this sequence is repeated about 6 to 50 times. 51–200 repeats occur in 'premutational' individuals (offspring at risk). Over 200 repeats results in full mutation and individuals are usually affected.
   d **True.**
   e **True.** The characteristic phenotype includes; elongated face and mandible, large ears, macrocephaly, soft skin and other tissues, macroorchidism, and mild short stature.

Laxova, R. (1994) Fragile X syndrome (Review). *Advances in Paediatrics* 41, 305–342.

1.42

   a **False.** High creatine phophokinase levels.
   b **False.** Low serum iron.
   c **True.**
   d **False.** It can be caused by all classes of antipsychotics. After full recovery one can cautiously use the same drug again, but generally it is best to use a different class of antipsychotic.
   e **True.** As a result of muscular rigidity.

Cookson, J., Crammer, J. and Heine, B. (1993) *The use of drugs in psychiatry*, 3rd edn. Gaskell, London, p. 66.

Questions

1.43

In the treatment of mania

	High	Med	Low
a Approximately two-thirds of patients show a good response to lithium salts within a 2 week period.	...	...	...
b Antipsychotics are first line treatments of choice for prophylaxis.	...	...	...
c Sodium valproate should be considered in those who have not responded to lithium or carbamazepine.	...	...	...
d Benzodiazepines are indicated for those patients who are not adequately sedated by antipsychotics.	...	...	...
e Double-blind trials have shown ECT to be superior to lithium for severe mania.	...	...	...

1.44

Stereotactic subcaudate tractotomy carried out for depression

a Has a good outcome in approximately 20% of cases.	...	...	...
b Causes seizures in approximately 10% of patients.	...	...	...
c Involves insertion of cadmium rods.	...	...	...
d Reduces the suicide rate to close to 1%.	...	...	...
e Is a treatment covered by Section 57 of the Mental Health Act (1983).	...	...	...

1.45

The following statements are true:

a In England children are not held criminally responsible until the age of 12.	...	...	...
b Sleep-walking is, for legal purposes, classed as a disease of the mind.	...	...	...
c A manslaughter (culpable homicide) charge, allows for a wide discretion in sentencing.	...	...	...
d Indecent exposure leads on to serious sexual assault in about 30% of cases.	...	...	...
e Shoplifters with a depressive illness usually make little effort to conceal their actions.	...	...	...

1.46

According to Jerome Frank the following are common factors necessary for successful psychotherapy:

a Unconditional positive regard.	...	...	...
b Emotional arousal.	...	...	...
c Instillation of hope.	...	...	...
d Regular weekly sessions.	...	...	...
e New information about the nature of the problem.	...	...	...

Answers

1.43

a **True.**

b **False.** Mood stabilizers such as lithium are recommended as first line.

c **True.**

d **True.**

e **True.**

Taylor, D. and Duncan, D. (1997) Doses of carbamazepine and sodium valproate in bipolar affective disorder. *Psychiatric Bulletin* 21(4), 221–223.

Cookson, J., Crammer, J. and Heine, B. (1993) *The use of drugs in psychiatry*, 3rd edn. Gaskell, London, pp. 87–92.

1.44

a **False.** Has a good outcome in more than 50% of cases.

b **False.** Less than 2%.

c **False.** Radioactive yttrium rods.

d **True.** From approximately 15% for depressive illnesses not treated surgically.

e **True.**

Bridges, P.K. *et al.* (1994) Psychosurgery: stereotactic subcaudate tractotomy. an indispensable treatment. *British Journal of Psychiatry* 165, 599–611.

1.45

a **False.** 10 years.

b **True.**

c **True.** Compared with a mandatory life sentence for murder.

d **False.** Most offenders do not re-offend. It rarely progresses to more serious sexual offending.

e **True.**

Gelder, M., Gath, D., Mayou, R., and Cowen, P. (eds.) (1996) *The Oxford textbook of psychiatry*, 3rd edn. Oxford University Press, Oxford, pp. 763–773.

1.46

a **False.** This is part of Rogerian theory.

b **True.**

c **True.**

d **False.**

e **True.**

Note: The other factors according to Frank are an intense confiding relationship with a helping person, a rationale that gives an account of the patient's problems and methods for their resolution, and providing an opportunity to experience some success during therapy and so give an increased sense of mastery.

Frank, J. D. (1996) In Bloch, S. (Ed.) *An introduction to the psychotherapies*, 3rd edn. Oxford University Press, Oxford, pp. 11–13.

Questions

1.47

	[Certainty]		
Gestalt therapy, as proposed by Perls, includes	High	Med	Low
a Dramatization.	...	...	...
b Transference.	...	...	...
c Group therapy.	...	...	...
d Games with rules.	...	...	...
e Emphasis on the here and now.	...	...	...

1.48

Cognitive therapy

a Is similar to Kelly's personal construct therapy.	...	...	...
b Involves anxiety management.	...	...	...
c Is as efficacious as antidepressants prescribed at therapeutic levels for recurrently depressed patients.	...	...	...
d Is as effective as maintenance medication in the prevention of relapse after an acute episode of depression.	...	...	...
e Is less effective as a treatment for depressive disorders than for anxiety or phobic disorders.	...	...	...

1.49

Drivers of Public Service or Heavy Goods Vehicles with a mental disorder in the UK

a Can hold a driving licence if suffering from mental impairment.	...	...	...
b Require a 1 year period of abstinence prior to renewal of a licence if previously dependent on alcohol.	...	...	...
c Can hold a driving licence if they are on regular antipsychotic medication.	...	...	...
d May drive after 6 months symptom free after any psychotic illness.	...	...	...
e Should have their licence refused or revoked if they lack insight into their condition.	...	...	...

Answers

1.47

a **True.**

b **False.** Transference is not encouraged.

c **True.** Gestalt is practised in group settings.

d **True.**

e **True.**

Brown, D. and Pedder, J. (1991) *Introduction to psychotherapy*, 2nd edn. Routledge, London, pp. 170–172.

1.48

a **True.** Personal construct therapy engages with patients to discover their maladaptive thinking about themselves and their environment.

b **True.** Along with cognitive restructuring and behavioural modification.

c **True.**

d **True.**

e **False.** It is more effective for depressive disorders.

Brown, D. and Pedder, J. (1991) *Introduction to psychotherapy*, 2nd edn. Routledge, London, pp. 177–179.

Blackburn, I.M. and Moore, R.G. (1997) Controlled acute and follow-up trial of cognitive therapy and pharmacotherapy in out-patients with recurrent depression. *British Journal of Psychiatry* 171, 328–334.

1.49

a **True.** Assuming it is of mild degree and the condition is stable.

b **False.** 3 years is the required period.

c **False.** They may, however, be allowed to hold a licence at the discretion of the DVLA if on treatment with an SSRI having recovered from an episode of depression and symptom free.

d **False.** At least 3 years off driving after which the patient should be symptom-free.

e **True.**

Taylor, J.F. (ed.) (1995) The Medical Commission on Accident Prevention. *Medical aspects of fitness to drive. a guide for medical practitioners*, 5th edn. HMSO, London, pp. 110–117.

Questions
1.50

The recovery of memories of childhood sexual abuse	High	Med	Low
a Should be actively pursued in adults with unexplained neurotic symptoms.	...	...	...
b Is facilitated by regression therapy.	...	...	...
c By adult patients should lead to mandatory reporting by the psychiatrist.	...	...	...
d Is also known as 'False memory syndrome'.	...	...	...
e Is facilitated by drug-assisted interviews.	...	...	...

[Certainty]

Answers

1.50

a **False.** The Royal College of Psychiatrists has recently issued a set of recommendations for good practice in treating patients with 'recovered memories' of childhood sexual abuse. The College advises against persuasive or suggestive psychotherapeutic techniques designed to unearth sexual abuse to which the patient has no memory and to question the historical accuracy of patients' recovered memories.

b **False.**

c **False.** But mandatory reporting is appropriate where children or adolescents spontaneously report current or recent abuse.

d **True.**

e **False.** Techniques such as regression therapy or drug-assisted interviews are of unproved effectiveness.

Royal College of Psychiatrists' Working Group on Reported Memories of Childhood Sexual Abuse. (1997) *Psychiatric Bulletin* 21(10), 663–665.

Pope, H.G. Jr (1998) Recovered memories of childhood sexual abuse. *British Medical Journal* 316, 488–489.

Paper 2: Questions

Basic science

2.1

The following distinguish a cohort from a case–control study: High Med Low

a A comparison group of controls are selected to resemble ...   .
   cases in a cohort study.

b In a cohort study exposure is measured before ...   .
   development of disease.

c Risk or incidence of disease can be measured directly in a ...   .
   case–control study.

d A cohort study begins with a defined population at risk. ...   .

e Cases are not selected in a cohort study but ascertained ...   .
   by a single examination of the population.

2.2

The odds ratio

a Estimates relative risk in prospective studies. ...   .

b Is useful in case–control studies. ...   .

c Is low when there is a probable association between ...   .
   groups.

d Should always be specified with the 95% confidence ...   .
   interval.

e Of a small sample will lead to a small confidence interval. ...   .

2.3

In the assessment of intelligence

a Intelligence quotient can be expressed as ...   .
   (chronological age) divided by (mental age) multiplied
   by 100.

b Original mental age scales were devised by Stanford. ...   .

c The Weschler Adult Intelligence Scale (WAIS) has ...   .
   performance and verbal subscales.

d The WAIS has high validity but low reliability. ...   .

e The Weschler Preschool and Primary Scale of ...   .
   Intelligence (WPPSI) is used for assessing intelligence in
   young children.

Paper 2: Answers

Basic science

2.1

a **False.** A comparison group (i.e. non-cases) are not selected but evolve naturally within a cohort study, whereas the investigator selects matched controls in the case–control study.

b **True.** Exposure is measured, reconstructed, or recollected after development of disease in a case–control study.

c **False.** This is only true for a cohort study. Case–control and prevalence studies estimate relative risk via the odds ratio.

d **True.** Whereas the population at risk is generally undefined in a case–control study.

e **False.** This is the method for a prevalence study. Continuous surveillance of the population yields cases in a cohort study, whereas the investigator selects cases from a pool of patients in the case control study.

Gelder, M., Gath, D., Mayou, R., and Cowen, P. (eds.) (1996) *The Oxford textbook of psychiatry*, 3rd edn. Oxford University Press, Oxford, p. 87.

2.2

a **False.** The odds ratio measures relative risk in retrospective studies, such as case–control studies. It helps compare two data sets (e.g. the relationship between schizophrenia and obstetric complications).

b **True.**

c **False.** The higher the odds ratio, the more likely there is to be an association between two grouping variables. For example, an odds ratio of 2 implies that the association is twice as likely to occur than chance would predict.

d **True.** This is conventional good practice.

e **False.** A small sample leads to a wide or big 95% confidence interval, indicating that caution in interpretation is needed.

Altman, D. G. (1991) *Practical statistics for medical research*. Chapman and Hall, London, pp. 266–271.

2.3

a **False.** Mental age divided by chronological age multiplied by 100.

b **False.** Binet was the originator of mental age scales at the beginning of the century. The Stanford–Binet is a widely used scale to assess intelligence.

c **True.**

d **False.** High validity and high reliability.

e **True.**

Puri, B. and Tyrer, P. (1992) *Sciences basic to psychiatry*. Churchill Livingstone, Edinburgh, pp. 290–291.

Questions
2.4

	[Certainty]		
Thyrotropin releasing factor (TRF)	High	Med	Low
a Causes lowering of mood when administered to normal subjects.	...	...	...
b When administered to patients with depressive illnesses, fails to cause a normal rise in TSH levels in at least 50% of cases.	...	...	...
c CSF levels have been found to be raised in patients with depressive illness.	...	...	...
d Normal circadian rhythm of release is altered in depressed patients.	...	...	...
e Causes release of TSH from the neurohypophysis.	...	...	...

2.5

Antidepressants which inhibit the re-uptake of serotonin include

a Venlafaxine.	...	...	...
b Nefazadone.	...	...	...
c Trazadone.	...	...	...
d Mianserin.	...	...	...
e Mirtazapine.	...	...	...

2.6

The following are correctly paired with their antidotes:

a Aspirin—activated charcoal.	...	...	...
b Paracetamol—methionine.	...	...	...
c Dextropropoxyphene—naltrexone.	...	...	...
d Diazepam—flumazenil.	...	...	...
e Lead—sodium calcium edetate.	...	...	...

2.7

The following statements are true:

a Sulpiride is an example of a dibenzodiazepine.	...	...	...
b Photosensitivity is more likely with phenothiazines than butyrophenones.	...	...	...
c Substituted benzamides specifically block D_2 receptors.	...	...	...
d Chloral hydrate and the cyclopyrrolones both act at GABA receptors.	...	...	...
e Trazodone should not be prescribed for those with glaucoma or prostatism.	...	...	...

Answers

2.4

a **False.** It has been found to elevate mood in normal subjects.

b **False.** Nearer to 25% therefore decreasing any clinical usefulness for diagnosis.

c **True.**

d **True.**

e **False.** TSH is secreted from the adenohypophysis.

Note: Problems with specificity and sensitivity limit the clinical utility of endocrine challenge tests in psychiatry.

Puri, B. and Tyrer, P. (1992) *Sciences basic to psychiatry*. Churchill Livingstone, Edinburgh, pp. 56–57.

2.5

a **True.** Serotonin (5HT) and noradrenaline (NA) reuptake blocker.

b **True.** $5HT_2$ and weak 5HT reuptake inhibitor.

c **False.** $5HT_2$ antagonist, antihistamine, and α_1 antagonist.

d **False.** $5HT_2$, α_1, α_2, and histamine$_1$ antagonist.

e **False.** $5HT_2$, $5HT_3$, histamine$_1$, and α_2 antagonist.

Stahl, S.M. (1997) *Psychopharmacology of antidepressants*. Martin Dunitz, London, pp. 61–79

2.6

a **False.** There is no specific antidote to aspirin poisoning but activated charcoal enhances elimination by reducing absorption.

b **True.** The other antidote is acetylcysteine or parvolex.

c **False.** Naloxone is the specific opioid antagonist, but remember it is short-acting. Naltrexone is an aid to relapse prevention in people previously opioid dependent.

d **True.** But advice should be sought, as adverse effects such as convulsions can occur.

e **True.** Useful in all heavy metal poisoning, especially lead.

British National Formulary. Chapter: Emergency treatment of poisoning.

2.7

a **False.** Sulpiride is a substituted benzamide. Clozapine is a dibenzodiazepine.

b **True.** Photosensitivity is relatively rare with butyrephenones.

c **True.** E.g. sulpiride.

d **True.** Chloral hydrate is a propanediol, zopiclone is a cyclopyrrolone.

e **False.** Has few antimuscarinic effects compared to other tricyclic antidepressants.

Puri, B. and Tyrer, P. (1992) *Sciences basic to psychiatry*. Churchill Livingstone, Edinburgh, pp. 133–137.

British National Formulary, Section 4.3.

Questions
2.8
[Certainty]

The following conditions display autosomal dominant inheritance:

	High	Med	Low
a Agenesis of the corpus callosum.	...	...	...
b Lesch–Nyhan syndrome.	...	...	...
c Rett's syndrome.	...	...	...
d Huntington's disease.	...	...	...
e Acute intermittent porphyria.	...	...	...

2.9
The following statements about genetic disorders are true:

	High	Med	Low
a In X-linked dominant inheritance, all male offspring of affected males will inherit the disorder.	...	...	...
b Edward's syndrome is caused by trisomy of chromosome 18.	...	...	...
c Approximately 4% of cases of Down's syndrome are caused by a translocation involving chromosome 21.	...	...	...
d Low lod scores (logarithm of the odds) indicate significant linkage of genes.	...	...	...
e The XYY syndrome is associated with above average height.	...	...	...

2.10
These syndromes and neuroanatomical locations are correctly paired:

	High	Med	Low
a Broca's aphasia—prefrontal cortex.	...	...	...
b Alexia without agraphia (pure word blindness)—left angular gyrus.	...	...	...
c Pure agraphia—Exner's area.	...	...	...
d Alexia with agraphia—auditory pathway to dominant temporal lobe.	...	...	...
e Transcortical aphasia—temporal–parietal regions.	...	...	...

2.11
Diencephalic lesions result in

	High	Med	Low
a Amnesia of Korsakoff type.	...	...	...
b Hypersomnia.	...	...	...
c Akinetic mutism.	...	...	...
d Constructional apraxia.	...	...	...
e Intractable pain.	...	...	...

Answers
2.8
    a **False.** Autosomal recessive or X-linked.
    b **False.** X-linked recessive condition characterized by hyperuricaemia and self-mutilation.
    c **False.** X-linked dominant (only reported in females).
    d **True.** A subcortical dementia.
    e **True.** A rare but important cause of psychiatric disturbance.

Puri, B. and Tyrer, P. (1992) *Sciences basic to psychiatry*. Churchill Livingstone, Edinburgh, pp. 157–159.

2.9
    a **False.** Males do not inherit an X chromosome from their fathers.
    b **True.** Characterized by severe mental retardation and skull, chest, and limb abnormalities.
    c **True.**
    d **False.** High lod scores (logarithm of the odds) indicate linkage of genes that are in close proximity to each other.
    e **True.** Occurs in 1 in 700 live male births. Slightly lower than average IQ scores.

Puri, B. and Tyrer, P. (1992) *Sciences basic to psychiatry*. Churchill Livingstone, Edinburgh, pp. 157–161, 172.

2.10
    a **True.**
    b **False.** Pure word blindness—left visual cortex and splenium of corpus callosum (area supplied by the posterior cerebral artery).
    c **True.** The foot of the second left frontal gyrus.
    d **False.** Alexia with agraphia—left angular gyrus.
    e **False.** Transcortical aphasia—damage to nerve connections (arcus fasiculus) between Broca's area and Wernicke's area, resulting in an inability to produce spontaneous speech but intact ability to repeat phrases.

Weller, M. and Eysenck, M. (1991) *The scientific basis of psychiatry*, 2nd edn. Saunders, Philadelphia, pp. 165–169.

2.11
    a **True.**
    b **True.**
    c **True.**
    d **False.** This usually occurs with parietal lobe lesions.
    e **True.** Thalamic lesions are associated with pain and sensory disorders.

Note: Diencephalic structures include thalamus, hypothalamus, subthalamus, and epithalamus. Hypothalamic lesions may result in polydipsia, polyuria, increase in body temperature, obesity, and disturbance of sexual function.

Puri, B. and Tyrer, P. (1992) *Sciences basic to psychiatry*. Churchill Livingstone, Edinburgh, p. 182.

Questions
2.12
[Certainty]

Long-term potentiation (LTP)   High   Med   Low

a Describes how memory recall is enhanced by learning by   ...   .
   meaning.
b Is another term for long-term memory.   ...   .
c Refers to the long lasting increase in the efficacy of a   ...   .
   specific set of synapses.
d Depends on the activation of the NMDA receptor.   ...   .
e Is associated with an increase in intracellular calcium   ...   .
   ions.

2.13

Regarding the neuronal action potential:

a The polarity of the voltage across the cell membrane   ...   .
   changes from positive to negative.
b Sodium influx precedes potassium influx into the cell.   ...   .
c Schwann cells help increase conduction velocity.   ...   .
d During the refractory period no further action potentials   ...   .
   can be elicited.
e Nerve fibres to muscle have the highest conduction   ...   .
   velocities of all excitable tissue.

2.14

The scalp recorded electroencephalogram (EEG)

a Records summated cortical cell action potentials.   ...   .
b Is abnormal in 15% of non-epileptic patients.   ...   .
c Show more abnormalities after sleep deprivation.   ...   .
d Shows more abnormalities with rhythmic auditory   ...   .
   stimulation.
e Shows more abnormalities with hypoventilation.   ...   .

Answers
2.12

  a **False.**

  b **False.**

  c **True.** If electrodes are implanted into specific pathways into the hippo-campus and short bursts of high frequency stimulation given, connections associated with that pathway are strengthened. This is termed LTP, which is thought to be a substrate of associative learning.

  d **True.**

  e **True.**

Kendell, R.E. and Zealley, A.K. (eds.) (1993) *Companion to psychiatric studies*, 5th edn. Churchill Livingstone, Edinburgh, pp. 157–158.

2.13

  a **False.** The voltage changes from around –60 mV to +35 mV across the neuronal membrane.

  b **False.** Sodium influx causes membrane depolarization, but repolarization occurs once the voltage-gated potassium channels are open, and potassium leaves the cell.

  c **True.** Insulating Schwann cells reduce axon capacitance, increasing con-duction velocity. A greater axon diameter reduces resistance which also improves conduction.

  d **False.** Initially this is so (the absolute refractory period) but later during the relative refractory period a suprathreshold stimulus will lead to an action potential.

  e **True.** 70–120 m s^{-1}, compared to cutaneous mechanoreceptors (25–70 m s^{-1}) and pain fibres (1 m s^{-1}).

Morgan, G. and Butler, S. (eds.) (1993) *Seminars in basic neurosciences*. Gaskell, London, pp. 45–48.

2.14

  a **False.** The EEG records the changing synaptic potential of cortical pyramidal neurones. The action potential is too short in comparison to show on the EEG.

  b **True.**

  c **True.**

  d **True.** In a similar way to the more often used photic stimulation.

  e **False.** Hyperventilation may be used to highlight abnormalities.

Puri, B. and Tyrer, P. (1992) *Sciences basic to psychiatry*. Churchill Livingstone, Edinburgh, pp. 62–64.

Laidlaw, J., Richens, A., and Chadwick, D. (1993) *A textbook of epilepsy*, 4th edn. Churchill Livingstone, London, pp. 291–294.

Questions

2.15

		[Certainty]	
The following statements are true:	High	Med	Low
a Bonding describes the formation of attachment of infant to mother.	...	...	...
b The concept of object permanence develops at around 8 months.	...	...	...
c Attachment formation continues into middle childhood.	...	...	...
d Secure attachments formed later may reverse the detrimental effects of early insecure attachment to mother.	...	...	...
e Children displaying 'ambivalent' reactions in the 'strange situation' are more likely to have a physically aggressive mother.	...	...	...

2.16

In human psychological development

a Infants do not develop selective attachments until after the age of 10 months.	...	...	...
b Smiling or crying by infants on reunion with mother is likely to indicate secure attachment.	...	...	...
c According to Bowlby's 'separation anxiety' protest is followed by detachment then despair.	...	...	...
d Winnicot suggests that transitional objects are used by the child in order to reduce anxiety.	...	...	...
e Gender identity is acquired at around 4 years of age.	...	...	...

2.17

The following are tests of frontal lobe function:

a Stroop Colour–Word Interference Test.	...	...	...
b Digit span.	...	...	...
c Verbal fluency.	...	...	...
d Wisconsin Card Sort test.	...	...	...
e Digit symbol substitution.	...	...	...

Answers

2.15

a **False.** Bonding refers to the attachment of mother to infant.

b **True.** Infants attain the concept that objects exist even although they may no longer be visible.

c **True.** Attachments continue to form throughout life.

d **True.**

e **False.** More likely to have an 'insensitive' mother.

Tantum, D. and Birchwood, M. (eds.) (1994) *Seminars in psychology and the social sciences.* Gaskell, London, pp. 151–165.

2.16

a **False.** Over 7 months.

b **True.**

c **False.** Protest and despair are followed by detachment.

d **True.** Such as a teddy bear.

e **False.** Usually acquired by 2 years.

Black, D. and Cottrell, D. (eds.) (1993) *Seminars in Child and Adolescent Psychiatry.* Gaskell, London, pp. 6–27.

2.17

a **True.** The Stroop test is comprised of a number of sub-components. One of these requires the subject to read a list of colours which are written in a disparate colour thereby creating an interference task.

b **False.** This is a subscale of the Wechsler Adult Intelligence Scale (WAIS) and is a measure of verbal intelligence.

c **True.** Verbal fluency is tested by asking the subject to think of as many words as he can beginning with various letters over usually one minute. This can also be done with categories, e.g. 'think of as many flowers as you can'. These tests are presumed to reflect frontal lobe function.

d **True.**

e **False.** This is a subscale of the Wechsler Adult Intelligence Scale (WAIS) and is a measure of performance IQ.

Tantum, D. and Birchwood, M. (eds.) (1994) *Seminars in psychology and the social sciences.* Gaskell, London, pp. 115–119, 134.

Gelder, M., Gath, D., Mayou, R., and Cowen, P. (eds.) (1996) *The Oxford textbook of psychiatry,* 3rd edn. Oxford University Press, Oxford, p. 319.

Questions
2.18

	[Certainty]		
In the personal construct theory	High	Med	Low
a Reality is objective.	...	...	...
b The Repertory Test or Grid is used.	...	...	...
c Constructs can be multidimensional.	...	...	...
d Humans are purely reactive.	...	...	...
e Schizophrenia is due to excessively loosened personal constructs.	...	...	...

2.19

Obedience to authority			
a Is enhanced if it is believed that the instructor has valid authority.	...	...	...
b Increases with increasing physical distance from the instructor or experimenter.	...	...	...
c Increases with increasing physical distance from a potential victim of those instructions.	...	...	...
d Is associated with classic studies carried out by Milliken.	...	...	...
e Can easily cause normal people to carry out potentially violent or antisocial acts.	...	...	...

2.20

Impulsive aggression			
a Is rarely seen in modern warfare.	...	...	...
b Is linked to low cerebral serotonin.	...	...	...
c Can be explained by poor parenting.	...	...	...
d Has been associated with a deficiency of the enzyme monoamine oxidase A.	...	...	...
e Is more common in men with schizophrenia.	...	...	...

Answers
2.18

a **False.** There is no objective reality, only alternative constructions from which to choose.

b **True.** Devised by George Kelly (1955) to assess an individual's constructs.

c **False.** Constructs are only dichotomous, according to Kelly.

d **False.** Humans constantly attempt to scientifically predict their environment.

e **True.**

Dinan, T.G. (1985) *Examination notes on the scientific basis of psychiatry.* Wright, Bristol, p. 92.

2.19

a **True.**

b **False.** Proximity of instructor increases compliance with commands.

c **True.**

d **False.** Milgram. Milliken was a physicist.

e **True.**

Note: The classic series of experiments by Milgram in the USA demonstrated various features that can cause normal subjects to comply with authority. The commission of violent acts by soldiers in war is a clear example of compliance with authority.

Puri, B. and Tyrer, P. (1992) *Sciences basic to psychiatry.* Churchill Livingstone, Edinburgh, p. 288.

2.20

a **True.** Occasionally, at times of long-term fear (e.g. the My Lai massacre) impulsive aggression occurs during industrialized warfare but it is not the rule.

b **True.** A low CSF 5-hydroxyidoleacetic acid (5HIAA, a metabolite of 5HT) is a concomitant to impaired impulse control.

c **False.** Controversial.

d **True.** MAO-A catalyses the oxidation of 5HT to 5HIAA in the raphe neurons. A stop codon mutation has been described in a large Dutch pedigree, but this is probably rare.

e **True.** About 50% of violence undertaken by male schizophrenics is directly attributable to positive symptoms (delusions) and possibly emerges late in the illness. The relationship between female schizophrenics and violence is less clear.

Genetics of Criminal and Antisocial Behaviour (1996) CIBA Foundation Symposium 194. Wiley, London.

Questions

2.21

	[Certainty]

Regarding neonatal social development:

	High	Med	Low
a Smiling becomes discriminatory after 3 months.	...	...	...
b Infants show a preference for the mother's face over other face-type configurations after a few months.	...	...	...
c Wide cheeks, short face, and large wide-set eyes have been shown to be most appealing to adults.	...	...	...
d The neonate has an internal representation of self.	...	...	...
e The neonate is not distressed at separation from the mother.	...	...	...

2.22

The following expressed emotion (EE) factors have been found to predict relapse in patients with schizophrenia

	High	Med	Low
a A low level of face-to-face contact with others in the home.	...	...	...
b Emotional overinvolvement with close relatives.	...	...	...
c Being actively ignored by close relatives.	...	...	...
d Inconsistent support from close relatives.	...	...	...
e Hostility from close relatives.	...	...	...

2.23

Hydrocephalus has a recognized association with

	High	Med	Low
a Adrenoleucodystrophy.	...	...	...
b Arnold–Chiari malformation.	...	...	...
c Subarachnoid haemorrhage.	...	...	...
d Alzheimer's disease.	...	...	...
e Pellagra.	...	...	...

Answers

2.21

a **True.** Early smiling is indiscriminate, but becomes more social in intent after 3 months. Thus, early smiling or orientating to stimuli give the appearance of social intent but can be elicited by a stranger.

b **False.** This develops after a few days. Early visual acuity (and hearing) is poor, but infants prefer to track face-type configurations from birth.

c **True.** This draws attention to the infant's face, and is part of the non-verbal care-eliciting behaviour upon which the infant's survival depends.

d **False.** Infants can imitate the facial expression of others, but this is not true imitation as the infant has no concept of self and other.

e **True.** The mother, or care-giver is made to feel the infant is aware of her and responds positively. However, this is not true attachment (see a, above).

Tantum, D. and Birchwood, M. (eds.) (1994) *Seminars in psychology and the social sciences.* Gaskell, London, pp. 153–155.

2.22

a **False.** Low level face-to-face contact and communication predicted poor outcome in depression, but was protective in schizophrenia.

b **True.** The three factors found to be important were critical comments, hostility, and emotional overinvolvement by close relatives.

c **False.** Vaughan and Leff found that a high level of EE (>35 hours per week contact) was a better predictor of relapse than non-compliance with medication. Also the robustness of EE as a predictor of relapse in schizophrenia has been confirmed across a range of cultures.

d **False.** However, neither c or d is particularly desirable.

e **True.**

Tantum, D. and Birchwood, M. (eds.) (1994) *Seminars in psychology and the social sciences.* Gaskell, London, pp. 251–255.

2.23

a **False.** This X-linked recessive condition is characterized by extensive myelin degeneration. Adrenal abnormalities are also seen.

b **True.** This is a spina bifida associated with elongated cerebellar tonsils, which protrude through the foramen magnum. A kinked medulla and hydrocephalus are present.

c **True.** A subarachnoid haemorrhage can lead to obstruction of CSF movement through the subarachnoid space or across arachnoid granulations.

d **True.** Not characteristic, but the loss of substance type associated with widened sulci (as seen in Alzheimer's) can cause hydrocephalus.

e **False.** Chronic nicotinic acid deficiency leads to pellagra, which can be summarized by the 'three Ds', i.e. diarrhoea; dermatitis; and depression. However, a variety of psychiatric problems can be seen, including mania and paranoia. Tryptophan is a precursor to nicotinic acid.

Morgan, G. and Butler, S. (eds.) (1993) *Seminars in basic neurosciences.* Gaskell, London, pp. 210–217.

Questions
2.24
[Certainty]

	High	Med	Low

The following statements regarding cerebral lesions and their sequelae are true:

a Utilization behaviour and palillalia are seen in frontal lobe disease.   ...   .

b Prosopagnosia and hemisomatognosia are seen in dominant temporal lobe disease.   ...   .

c Agraphia is a feature of Gerstmann's syndrome.   ...   .

d Posterior cerebral artery occlusion results in alexia without agraphia.   ...   .

e Personality change is rare after subarachnoid haemorrhage. ...   .

2.25
Regarding demyelinating diseases:

a Central pontine myelinosis is most commonly seen in chronic alcoholism.   ...   .

b Axonal degeneration is usually present.   ...   .

c Multiple sclerosis commonly presents as a psychotic illness.   ...   .

d Disorders of sphingolipid metabolism may be a cause.   ...   .

e Schilder's disease is also known as diffuse cerebral sclerosis.   ...   .

Clinical

2.26
Regarding the development of depressive illness after stroke:

a Depression is thought to be more common following a right rather than a left hemisphere lesion.   ...   .

b Depression is more common following a posterior lesion than an anterior one.   ...   .

c Any depression is strongly associated with the degree of intellectual impairment.   ...   .

d A family history of depression contributes to the risk of depression after stroke.   ...   .

e Tricyclic antidepressants should not be used in depression after stroke.   ...   .

Answers
2.24

   a **True.** Utilization behaviour is, for example, writing whenever a pen comes within grasp. Palilalia is the repetition of sentences or phrases.
   b **False.** The non-dominant hemisphere. Hemisomatonosia is neglect of one side of the body.
   c **True.** Also includes dyscalculia, finger agnosia, and left–right disorientation.
   d **True.** Inability to read.
   e **False.** Personality changes occur in approximately 20% of cases.

Puri, B. and Tyrer, P. (1992) *Sciences basic to psychiatry*. Churchill Livingstone, Edinburgh, pp. 181–184.

2.25

   a **True.** This is a rare and fatal demyelinating condition.
   b **False.** Histologically, there is periaxial demyelination with preservation of axons.
   c **False.** Psychosis is rarely a presenting feature.
   d **True.** Examples include Niemann–Pick disease, Gaucher's disease, and Tay–Sachs disease.
   e **True.** Also known as encephalitis periaxalia diffusa.

Puri, B. and Tyrer, P. (1992) *Sciences basic to psychiatry*. Churchill Livingstone, Edinburgh, pp. 190–192.

Clinical

2.26

   a **False.** It is claimed that strokes involving the anterior part of the left hemisphere are particularly associated with depression. The evidence for this is not conclusive.
   b **False.** Statistically an anterior infarct is more often associated with depression than a posterior lesion.
   c **False.**
   d **True.**
   e **False.** Drugs should be given cautiously as side effects are frequent in this population. Although some tricyclic antidepressants are relatively contraindicated after myocardial infarction, no such caution is required post-stroke. Prior to treatment an ECG and blood pressure monitoring would be judicious.

Astrom, M. *et al.* (1993) Major depression in stroke patients: a 3 year longitudinal study. *Stroke* 24, 976–982.

Gelder, M., Gath, D., Mayou, R., and Cowen, P. (eds.) (1996) *The Oxford textbook of psychiatry*, 3rd edn. Oxford University Press, Oxford, pp. 330–331

Questions
2.27

	[Certainty]		
Deliberate self-poisoning with paracetamol	High	Med	Low
a Is a problem in most European countries.	...	...	...
b Is the most common drug for poisoning in the UK.	...	...	...
c Is the cause of approximately 15 deaths per year in the UK.	...	...	...
d May be made less harmful by the use of tablet blister-packs.	...	...	...
e Results in the hepatorenal syndrome.	...	...	...

2.28

Depressive disorder			
a With a seasonal pattern is usually associated with anorexia and insomnia.	...	...	...
b Is associated with low cortisol secretion which returns to normal levels on recovery from depression.	...	...	...
c Left untreated has a median length of duration of one year.	...	...	...
d Is associated with frontal lobe cerebral blood flow abnormalities.	...	...	...
e Has a recognized association with cancer.	...	...	...

2.29

The following statements are true:			
a Schizophrenia when defined by nuclear or Schneiderian symptoms varies greatly across different parts of the world.	...	...	...
b Obstetric complications are associated with a greater than expected risk of subsequently developing schizophrenia.	...	...	...
c Schneiderian first rank symptoms are required for an ICD 10 diagnosis of schizophrenia.	...	...	...
d It is established that marital schism and or skew are aetiologically significant in the development of schizophrenia.	...	...	...
e Structural brain abnormalities are now generally accepted to be associated with chronic schizophrenia.	...	...	...

Answers
2.27

 a **True.** The problem is not restricted to the UK.
 b **True.**
 c **False.** More than 10 times this number.
 d **True.** Hawton has suggested this may reduce the quantity of drug consumed.
 e **True.**

Hawton, K. *et al*. (1996) Paracetamol self-poisoning—characteristics, prevention and harm reduction. *British Journal of Psychiatry* 168, 43–48.

2.28

 a **False.** Characteristically associated with hyperphagia and hypersomnia.
 b **False.** It is associated with high cortisol secretion which returns to normal levels on recovery from depression. An abnormal dexamethasone suppression test (DST) is also described, as well as abnormal responses to challenges by various other hormones.
 c **True.** This is also true for mania.
 d **True.** Positron emission tomography (PET) has shown decreased glucose metabolism in frontal regions (hypofrontality).
 e **True.**

Kendell, R.E. and Zealley, A.K. (eds.) (1993) *Companion to psychiatric studies*, 5th edn. Churchill Livingstone, Edinburgh, pp. 427–453.

2.29

 a **False.** The International Pilot Study of Schizophrenia (IPSS) showed schizophrenia to be present in many different countries. When analysed by 'core', 'nuclear' or PSE 'Catego S+' criteria, the incidence of schizophrenia is remarkably consistent across different countries.
 b **True.** The odds ratio is approximately 2 by international meta-analysis.
 c **False.**
 d **False.**
 e **True.**

Kendell, R.E. and Zealley, A.K. (eds.) (1993) *Companion to psychiatric studies*, 5th edn. Churchill Livingstone, Edinburgh, pp. 397–423.

World Health Organization (1992) *Tenth revision of the International Classification of Disease (ICD 10)*. WHO, Geneva.

Questions

2.30

The following help distinguish schizotypal disorder from schizoid personality disorder:

[Certainty]

High   Med   Low

a Excessive preoccupation with fantasy.

b Poor rapport.

c A first degree relative with schizophrenia.

d Odd speech and appearance.

e Lack of close friends.

2.31

Shoplifting

a Is a predominantly male activity.

b Results in less than 5% of culprits being referred for psychiatric assessment.

c In psychiatrically disturbed patients most often attracts the diagnosis of mental handicap/learning difficulty.

d By the majority of females is a recidivist activity.

e Is a recognized diagnosis in ICD 10.

2.32

Regarding driving and psychiatric disorder:

a The licence holder is obliged to inform the DVLA as soon as they become aware of a disorder likely to affect their driving.

b The doctor should not breach confidentiality by informing the DVLA without the consent of the patient.

c Driving should cease for one year following a schizophrenic episode requiring hospitalization.

d Driving is not permitted with the onset of dementia.

e Driving should cease for 6 months following evidence of cannabis use.

Answers
2.30

  a **False.** Seen in both.

  b **False.** Poor empathy and a constricted affect can be found in both.

  c **True.** A genetic link between schizotypy, but not schizoid disorder, and schizophrenia has been documented.

  d **True.** Part of schizotypy, along with magical thinking; suspiciousness; obsessionality; and transient quasi-psychotic symptoms.

  e **False.** Not distinguishing, but perhaps more characteristic of schizoid disorder.

World Health Organization (1992) *Tenth revision of the International Classification of Disease (ICD 10)*, WHO, Geneva, pp. 95–7 and 203–4.

2.31

  a **False.** Unlike most other crimes, the majority of shoplifters are female (~80%).

  b **True.** Approximately 2%.

  c **False.** One third suffer from 'neuroses, psychosomatic disorders or compulsive behaviour', the rest from diagnoses such as personality disorders (17%), psychoses (15%), mental handicap (11%), organic disorders (5%), and alcohol or drug problems (3%).

  d **False.** One in ten of all shoplifters are thought to be recidivists (repeat offenders).

  e **False.**

Sims, A. (1988) *Symptoms in the mind. an introduction to descriptive psychopathology*. Ballière Tindall, London, pp. 268.

2.32

  a **True.**

  b **False.** This is possible if the doctor feels that the safety of others is at stake.

  c **False.** Six months.

  d **False.** If the dementia is mild, the patient may be permitted to drive if no significant disorientation is present and there is retention of insight and judgement.

  e **True.** Twelve months in the case of other drugs if there is evidence of dependency or abuse.

Taylor, J.F. (Ed.) (1995).The Medical Commission on Accident Prevention. *Medical aspects of fitness to drive. a guide for medical practitioners*, 5th edn. HMSO, London, pp. 110–117.

Questions
2.33

The following statements are true:

	High	Med	Low
a *Vorbeireden* is pathognomonic of Ganser syndrome.	...	...	...
b Anti-obsessional effects of 5HT re-uptake blockade take the same time as antidepressant effects to become apparent.	...	...	...
c According to ICD 10, the diagnosis of panic disorder requires the individual to have experienced at least 4 episodes of panic within a 2 week period.	...	...	...
d Most neurotic children become neurotic adults.	...	...	...
e During childhood, boys are more likely to suffer from 'neurosis' than girls.	...	...	...

2.34

In transsexualism

a The gender identity problem usually develops at or after puberty.	...	...	...
b The genitalia are often repugnant to the transsexual.	...	...	...
c A candidate for reassignment surgery should see a psychiatrist for at least 2 years prior to surgery.	...	...	...
d There is an approximately equal sex ratio of those affected.	...	...	...
e There is usually a low libido.	...	...	...

2.35

The following may be useful in the treatment of depression:

a A combination of fluoxetine and tranylcypromine.	...	...	...
b Pumpkin seeds.	...	...	...
c Sulpiride.	...	...	...
d Tri-iodothyronine.	...	...	...
e Diazepam.	...	...	...

Answers

2.33

a **False.** *Vorbeireden* (approximate answers) can occur in organic brain disease.

b **False.** Anti-obsessional effects of 5HT re-uptake blockade can take at least 4 weeks to become apparent.

c **False.** At least three episodes of panic within a 3 week period.

d **False.** Most neurotic children become normal adults.

e **True.** Although this pattern reverses after adolescence.

Kendell, R.E. and Zealley, A.K. (eds.) (1993) *Companion to Psychiatric Studies*, 5th edn. Churchill Livingstone, Edinburgh, pp. 485–515.

World Health Organization (1992) *Tenth revision of the International Classification of Disease (ICD 10)*. WHO, Geneva.

2.34

a **False.** Almost invariably a gender identity problem is reported from childhood.

b **True.** Most aspects of the anatomic sex are distasteful and inappropriate to the true transsexual, particularly the primary and secondary sexual characteristics.

c **False.** To establish the diagnosis the preoccupation with the gender identity problem should have been present for at least 2 years. Early surgery is ill-advised.

d **False.** Males outnumber females by roughly 3 : 1, but as many as eight times more males seek treatment.

e **True.** There is often co-existing anxiety or personality disturbance, but the transsexualism should not be part of another mental disorder (e.g. delusional disorder).

American Psychiatric Association (1987) *Diagnostic and statistical manual* DSM-IIIR, pp. 74–76.

2.35

a **False.** Although a combination of antidepressants can be valuable in resistant depression, using an SSRI and an MAOI should be avoided due to the risk of inducing the serotonin syndrome (particularly with the two drugs mentioned).

b **True.** 200 g of pumpkin seeds contains about 1 g of natural tryptophan, and had been used when tryptophan was unavailable.

c **True.** An equivalent efficacy to amitriptyline has been shown.

d **True.** Tri-iodothyronine augmentation of antidepressants has been demonstrated to be effective, especially in rapid cycling disorder. Subclinical hypothyroidism can lead to depression.

e **False.** Specifically advised against in the *British National Formulary*.

Bazire, S. (1994) *Psychotropic drug directory*, pp. 18–22.

Questions
2.36

In the treatment of alcohol problems

	High	Med	Low
a Doses of chlordiazepoxide and diazepam are approximately equivalent.	...	...	...
b Acamprosate is not recognized as an effective anti-craving agent.	...	...	...
c Disulfiram is available in soluble form.	...	...	...
d Calcium carbimide is a useful alternative in patients who have adverse reactions to disulfiram.	...	...	...
e On considering assisted withdrawal, benzodiazepines should be given before the breath or blood alcohol level has fallen to zero.	...	...	...

2.37

Tardive dyskinesia

a Is more common in men than women after long-term antipsychotic medication.	...	...	...
b Affects 5% of chronic users of antipsychotic medication.	...	...	...
c Is more likely in those with an organic brain disorder.	...	...	...
d Occurs in psychotic patients who have never taken antipsychotic medication.	...	...	...
e Usually improves when antipsychotics are withdrawn.	...	...	...

2.38

Dexamphetamine sulphate

a Is used in the treatment of catalepsy.	...	...	...
b Is used in children in the treatment of refractory hyperkinetic states.	...	...	...
c Is contraindicated in patients with hypertension.	...	...	...
d Is helpful in hyperkinetic disorder associated with Gilles de la Tourette syndrome.	...	...	...
e Is associated with growth retardation in children.	...	...	...

Answers
2.36

    a **False.** 5 mg diazepam = 15 mg chlordiazepoxide.

    b **False.** Large randomized controlled trials have shown abstinence of 20% of subjects for up to 1 year.

    c **True.** Therefore can enhance compliance in conjunction with the 'partnership' approach.

    d **True.**

    e **True.** Otherwise the risk of convulsions is greatly increased. Not doing so may have fatal results.

British National Formulary, Sections 4.1, 4.10,

Chick, J. (1996) Medication in the treatment of alcohol dependence. *Advances in Psychiatric Treatment* 2, 249–257.

2.37

    a **False.** More common in females.

    b **False.** Approximately 20%.

    c **True.**

    d **True.**

    e **False.** Characteristically worsens on withdrawal. An increase in the drug will transiently alleviate symptoms, though in the long term may make the problem even worse. The best strategy is to routinely monitor for extrapyramidal side effects and make sure one is prescribing the minimum dose of antipsychotic required to control symptoms.

Kendell, R.E. and Zealley, A.K. (eds.) (1993) *Companion to psychiatric studies*, 5th edn. Churchill Livingstone, Edinburgh, p. 823.

2.38

    a **False.** Used in the narcolepsy cataplexy syndrome. Delays the onset of rapid eye movement (REM) sleep which subjects with this syndrome rapidly fall into.

    b **True.**

    c **True.**

    d **False.** It will exacerbate tics.

    e **True.** Regular monitoring of height and weight recommended. Discontinuous treatment or 'drug holidays' have been suggested.

British National Formulary, Section 4.5

Questions

2.39   [Certainty]

Social phobias	High	Med	Low
a Include phobias of excretion.	...	...	...
b Include phobias of vomiting.	...	...	...
c Are more common in women.	...	...	...
e Should be treated by cognitive behavioural therapy.	...	...	...
d Are more commonly associated with alcohol abuse than other phobias.	...	...	...

2.40

In senile dementia of the Alzheimer type

	High	Med	Low
a The overall course is steady and smoothly progressive.	...	...	...
b Death is usually within 10–15 years of onset.	...	...	...
c Extrapyramidal symptoms are uncommon.	...	...	...
d Epilepsy affects less than 20% of cases.	...	...	...
e Changes resembling the Kluver–Bucy syndrome rarely occur.	...	...	...

2.41

Agenesis of the corpus callosum

	High	Med	Low
a Is compatible with normal functioning.	...	...	...
b Is often associated with epilepsy.	...	...	...
c Occurs postnatally.	...	...	...
d Is part of the Aicardi syndrome.	...	...	...
e Is associated with learning disability in about 40% of cases.	...	...	...

Answers
2.39

a **True.** Excessive anxiety is experienced in situations where the person may be observed and could be criticised. Avoidance behaviour is common. Phobias of excretion and vomiting are discrete social phobias.

b **True.** Fear that they themselves or others will vomit in a public place.

c **False.** Equally common in men and women.

d **True.** This is the psychological treatment of choice. Other psychological therapies (e.g. psychodynamic) and drug therapies (e.g. benzodiazepines, beta-blockers, antidepressants) may help.

e **True.**

Gelder, M., Gath, D., Mayou, R., and Cowen, P. (eds.) (1996) *The Oxford textbook of psychiatry*, 3rd edn. Oxford University Press, Oxford, pp. 171–173.

2.40

a **True.** Distinguishing it from other forms of dementia such as multi-infarct type.

b **False.** Usually 5–7 years.

c **False.** They occur in up to two-thirds of patients.

d **False.** Affects around 75%.

e **False.** The Kluver–Bucy syndrome includes symptoms such as hyperorality, hyperphagia, and apathy. Similar symptoms have been noted to occur in up to 75% of patients with Alzheimer's disease.

Lishman, W.A. (1998) *Organic psychiatry*, 3rd edn. Blackwell Science, Oxford, pp. 437–439.

2.41

a **True.** Often an incidental radiological finding.

b **True.** Anywhere from a quarter to two-thirds of cases present with fits.

c **False.** The callosum forms early in fetal life, but continues growing over the first 4 years and myelinates predominantly after birth.

d **True.** This is a rare developmental syndrome almost invariably affecting girls, comprising of a triad of callosal agenesis; infantile spasms; and ocular abnormalities such as chorioretinal lacunae.

e **True.** Often in the context of a more widespread neuropsychiatric disorder.

Lassonde, M and Jeeves, M. (eds.) (1994) Callosal agenesis. In *Advances in behavioural biology*. Plenum Press, New York.

Taylor, M. and David, A.S. (1998) Agenesis of the corpus callosum: a UK series of 56 cases. *Journal of Neurology, Neurosurgery and Psychiatry*.

Questions
2.42

	[Certainty]		
The following are more common in Pick's disease than in Creutzfeld–Jacob disease (CJD):	High	Med	Low
a Females affected more than males.	...	...	...
b A normal electroencephalogram (EEG).	...	...	...
c Atrophy of the temporal lobes.	...	...	...
d Rapid progression of dementia.	...	...	...
e Status spongiosis appearance of the brain.	...	...	...

2.43

The following are associated with subcortical dementia:

	High	Med	Low
a Human immunodeficiency virus (HIV) infection.	...	...	...
b Progressive supranuclear palsy.	...	...	...
c Multiple sclerosis.	...	...	...
d Alzheimer's disease.	...	...	...
e Hypothyroidism.	...	...	...

2.44

Cannabis

	High	Med	Low
a Commonly causes hallucinations.	...	...	...
b Causes similar adverse cognitive effects as chronic alcohol abuse.	...	...	...
c Dependence is rare among those who regularly use the drug.	...	...	...
d Contains as its active ingredient Δ_9-tetrahydrocannabinol.	...	...	...
e Use in adolescents is not associated with progression to use of opiates.	...	...	...

Answers

2.42

a **True.** Twice as many females are affected.

b **True.** Biphasic/triphasic waves seen in CJD.

c **True.** So called 'knife blade' atrophy which spares the posterior aspects of the temporal lobes.

d **False.** Rapid progression of dementia can occur in CJD which is said to have a mortality rate of 50% within the first 9 months of diagnosis.

e **False.** Status spongiosis appearance occurs in CJD.

Lishman, W.A. (1998) *Organic psychiatry*, 3rd edn. Blackwell Science, Oxford, pp. 461–462, 473–478.

2.43

a **True.**

b **True.** Progressive supranuclear palsy is an akinetic rigid syndrome with opthalmoplegia which responds poorly to L-dopa.

c **False.**

d **False.**

e **True.**

Note: Subcortical dementia refers to a clinical entity characterized by slowness of cognition, memory disturbances, visuospatial abnormalities, and alterations in mood and affect. Aphasia, agnosia, and apraxia are absent or occur late. Progressive multifocal leukoencephalopathy (PML) is caused by a papovavirus infection in an immunocompromised host, and leads to a rapid relentless dementia for which there is no known treatment.

Cummings, J. L. (1986) Subcortical dementia: neurophysiology, neuropsychiatry and pathophysiology. *British Journal of Psychiatry* 149, 682–697.

2.44

a **False.**

b **False.** Long-term heavy cannabis users are not as cognitively impaired as chronic alcoholics but are impaired compared to non-cannabis users.

c **False.** Dependence is the most prevalent risk of regular cannabis use, affecting up to half of those who use it daily.

d **True.**

e **False.** The use of tobacco and alcohol is said to typically precede the use of cannabis, which in turn precedes the use of hallucinogens and opiates.

Note: Cannabis use and its psychiatric sequelae are a controversial area.

Gelder, M., Gath, D., Mayou, R., and Cowen, P. (eds.) (1996) *The Oxford textbook of psychiatry*, 3rd edn. Oxford University Press, Oxford, pp. 473–474.

Hall, W. and Solowij, N. (1997) Long-term cannabis use and mental health. *British Journal of Psychiatry* 171, 107–108.

Questions
2.45

Guardianship under the Mental Health Act confers the
following powers

	High	Med	Low
a The patient is deemed financially incapable.	...	...	...
b The patient is required to live at a place specified by the guardian.	...	...	...
c That access to the patient must be given to any registered medical practitioner.	...	...	...
d The patient is required to attend at a specified place for medical treatment.	...	...	...
e The patient can be removed from his residence against his or her will.	...	...	...

2.46

Phenylketonuria

a Has an incidence of 1 in 2000 births in the UK.	...	...	...
b Is caused by defective or absent DOPA decarboxylase enzyme.	...	...	...
c May be detected soon after birth by the Guthrie test.	...	...	...
d Requires that all phenylalanine be excluded from the diet.	...	...	...
e Sufferers should continue a restrictive diet at least into their teenage years.	...	...	...

2.47

In Gilles de la Tourette's syndrome

a Onset is rare before the age of 11.	...	...	...
b Males are affected 6 times more commonly than females.	...	...	...
c Mental coprolalia is said to be more common than overt coprolalia.	...	...	...
d Massed practice involves encouraging the subject to perform simultaneous incompatible movements.	...	...	...
e Haloperidol has been shown to be more beneficial than diazepam in treatment studies.	...	...	...

Answers
2.45

a **False.** A receiver (England and Wales), or curator bonis (Scotland) can be appointed to manage the affairs of the incapable adult.

b **True.**

c **True.**

d **True.** b, c and d are the three powers of guardianship, but there is no legal authority for detention or the use of force.

e **False.** Section 47 of the National Assistance Act can be so used if the patient is a danger to him or herself (i.e. mental disorder not essential).

Jacoby, R. and Oppenheimer, C. (eds.) (1991) *Psychiatry in the elderly*. Oxford Medical Publications, Oxford, p. 533.

2.46

a **False.** 1 in 14 000

b **False.** The enzyme at fault is phenylalanine hydroxylase.

c **True.**

d **False.** As phenylalanine is an essential amino acid a very small amount is required to be included in the diet.

e **True.**

Kendell, R.E. and Zealley, A.K. (eds.) (1993) *Companion to psychiatric studies*, 5th edn. Churchill Livingstone, Edinburgh, p. 632.

2.47

a **False.** The onset is usually at 5–8 years, but can be up to 16 years.

b **False.** 3 times as common in males.

c **True.**

d **False.** Massed practice involves repeating the movements/tics/obscenities as much as possible in an attempt to reduce them. Habit reversal involves performing simultaneous incompatible movements to reduce unwanted movements.

e **True.**

Lishman, W.A. (1998) *Organic psychiatry*, 3rd edn. Blackwell Science, Oxford, pp. 680–687.

Questions
2.48
[Certainty]

Cognitive behavioural therapy for moderate depressive illnesses	High	Med	Low
a Is less effective than tricyclic antidepressants in socially disadvantaged groups.	...	...	...
b Is most useful in those clearly showing negative automatic thoughts.	...	...	...
c Is not influenced by the educational level of the patient.	...	...	...
d Has a better outcome if the patient complies with homework tasks.	...	...	...
e Has been shown to be as effective as tricyclic antidepressants in several trials.	...	...	...

2.49

Correct associations are			
a Gestalt therapy—Bion.	...	...	...
b Therapeutic community—Main.	...	...	...
c T-groups—Yalom.	...	...	...
d Primal therapy—Perls.	...	...	...
e Cognitive analytic therapy—Ryle.	...	...	...

Answers
2.48

a **False.** There is no difference between social groups.

b **False.** The presence or absence of particular cognitive errors does not seem to have any bearing on outcome.

c **True.**

d **True.**

e **True.**

Moorey, S. (1996) Cognitive behaviour therapy for whom? *Advances in Psychiatric Treatment* 2, 17–23

2.49

a **False.** Fritz Perls devised gestalt therapy, usually undertaken in groups and concentrating on the 'here and now' rather than the transference.

b **True.** The term 'therapeutic community' was coined by Main, after the Second World War. He went on to found the Cassel Hospital.

c **False.** Although Yalom is well known for outlining important therapeutic factors in groups, it is Carl Rodgers who devised T-groups and later encounter groups.

d **False.** Arthur Janov wrote *The Primal Scream* and concentrated on the psychic trauma of childbirth.

e **True.** A recent hybrid of dynamic, cognitive, and personal construct therapy. A brief intervention perhaps particularly useful in anorexia nervosa.

Brown, D. and Pedder, J. (1991) *Introduction to psychotherapy*, 2nd edn. Routledge, London, pp. 151–178.

Questions
2.50

Regarding group psychotherapy:

a The leader should encourage transference by not   ...   .
   disclosing anything personal.

b It is the most common form of psychotherapy available   ...   .
   in the NHS.

c The instillation of dependency is a curative factor.   ...   .

d The concept of pairing involves a new leader or idea   ...   .
   bringing salvation to the group.

e Foulkes has been influential in its development in the UK. ...   .

Answers
2.50

a **False.** Transference will develop and should be interpreted, but equally the therapist will comment on countertransference. Patients benefit from a therapist being open and having the confidence to express him- or herself.

b **True.** A commitment to the group, sufficient ego-strength, and motivation for insight are thought to be prerequisites. Group therapy is probably cheaper than individual forms of psychotherapy. However, there is little outcome-based research.

c **False.** Yalom listed 12 'curative' factors important in group psychotherapy, including the instillation of hope. These make an easy MCQ target! The culture of dependency, assuming the leader will provide solutions, is one of Bion's basic assumptions of groups.

d **True.** The encouraging or hoping for a coupling of individuals which could lead to the birth of a person or idea that would provide salvation is another of Bion's basic assumptions of group culture. This attitude has been likened to the institution of aristocracy, and the Oedipus complex.

e **True.** Foulkes concentrated on analysis through and of the group, was instrumental in setting up the Institute of Group Analysis, and started the *Journal of Group Analysis*.

Brown, D. and Pedder, J. (1991) *Introduction to psychotherapy*, 2nd edn. Routledge, London, pp. 118–136.

Paper 3: Questions

Basic science

3.1

In epidemiology and research design   High   Med   Low

a Point prevalence can be described as incidence ×
   chronicity.

b The age of subjects is a potential confounding variable.

c The power of a test does not measure the likelihood of
   rejecting the null hypothesis.

d A type II error is the probability of detecting a significant
   difference when treatments are equally effective and is
   therefore a false positive.

e The attributable risk measures the importance of a risk
   factor in aetiology.

3.2

According to Liddle's classification of schizophrenia

a The psychomotor poverty syndrome is associated with
   underactivity in the dominant parietal lobe.

b The disorganization syndrome is characterized by
   deluded thinking.

c The disorganization syndrome is associated with excessive
   activity in the non-dominant anterior cingulate cortex.

d The reality distortion syndrome is associated with
   underactivity in the non-dominant medial temporal lobe.

e The classification was based on a factor analysis of
   cerebral blood flow patterns.

Paper 3: Answers

Basic science

3.1

a **True.** The point prevalence is the proportion of people suffering from an illness at a given point in time divided by the population at risk.

b **True.** A confounder is a variable which affects other variables in calculating measurements.

c **False.** The greater the power of a study, the better the chances of rejecting an incorrect null hypothesis.

d **False.** The possibility of not detecting a significant difference when there really is an important difference.

e **True.** The attributable risk is the incidence in a population which is exposed to a risk factor minus the incidence in a non-exposed population.

Puri, B. and Tyrer, P. (1992) *Sciences basic to psychiatry*. Churchill Livingstone, Edinburgh. pp 266–267, 269–274.

3.2

a **False.** The psychomotor poverty syndrome was linked to an underactivity in the dominant dorsolateral prefrontal cortex, a region maximally activated in normal subjects during self-generated mental functioning. The syndrome consists of poverty of speech, flatness of affect, and decreased spontaneous movement.

b **False.** The disorganisation syndrome is characterised by thought disorder and inappropriate (not blunted) affect.

c **True.** This area is implicated in attention tasks that involve the suppression of inappropriate mental activity.

d **False.** Associated with increased activity in the dominant medial temporal lobe. Normally this region is concerned with internal monitoring. The reality distortion syndrome is characterised by hallucinations and delusions.

e **True.** This was an important study because the classification was not descriptively but empirically based.

Liddle, P.F. *et al.* (1992) Patterns of cerebral blood flow in schizophrenia. *British Journal of Psychiatry* 160, 179–186.

Puri, B.K. (1995) *Saunder's pocket essentials of psychiatry*. Saunders, Philadelphia, p. 35.

Questions

3.3

	[Certainty]		
The following psychiatric instruments are self-rating scales:	High	Med	Low
a Hamilton Depression Rating Scale.	...	...	...
b Global Assessment Scale.	...	...	...
c Brief Psychiatric Rating Scale.	...	...	...
d Eating Attitudes Test.	...	...	...
e Minnesota Multiphasic Personality Inventory.	...	...	...

3.4

Male rhesus monkeys
   a Reared by mother are more aggressive than those reared   ...   .
     in peer groups.
   b Reared in restricted environments show deficiencies in   ...   .
     mounting behaviour that last into adulthood.
   c Reared in heterosexual groups show more aggressive   ...   .
     behaviour than those reared in same-sex groups.
   d Show more rough play than females, even in mixed-sex   ...   .
     groups.
   e Exhibit similar behaviours as those female rhesus   ...   .
     monkeys exposed *in utero* to exogenous male hormones.

3.5

Sociologist Ivan Illyich
   a Wrote *The myth of mental illness*.   ...   .
   b Described 'social iatrogenesis' whereby health policies   ...   .
     encouraged individual dependency and result in
     ill-health.
   c Viewed modern medicine as an all-enveloping   ...   .
     bureaucracy created by the state.
   d Advocated the removal of the exclusive right of doctors   ...   .
     to practice medicine.
   e Supported the demystification of medicine and an   ...   .
     increase in individual responsibility.

3.6

The following are correct associations:
   a Thorndike—social learning theory.   ...   .
   b Hawthorne—influence of social interaction of subject   ...   .
     and observer upon response.
   c Wolpe—law of effect.   ...   .
   d Bandura—systematic desensitization.   ...   .
   e Milgram—obedience with authority.   ...   .

Answers
3.3

   a **False.** Widely used observer rating scale, usually 17 or 21 items, not to be used as a diagnostic instrument.
   b **False.** Evaluates social functioning and severity of symptoms.
   c **False.** Frequently used 18-item measure of psychotic symptoms and psychopathology.
   d **True.** Self-report on eating behaviour.
   e **True.** This questionnaire has been validated on patients not normally given a 'personality profile'.

Buckey, P.F., Bird, J. and Harrison, G. (1995) *Examination notes in psychiatry*, 3rd edn. Butterworth-Heinemann, Oxford, pp. 6–7.

3.4

   a **False.** Male rhesus monkeys reared by the mother show competent sex behaviour and low levels of aggression, but infants reared in peer groups tend to be aggressive.
   b **True.**
   c **True.** It is thought that males occupy only dominant positions in mixed-sex groups, whilst in same-sex groups they are both dominant and subordinate.
   d **True.** Female rhesus monkeys show less rough play than males in mixed-sex groups, and particularly in same-sex groups.
   e **True.** The social conditions of rearing are also important, as illustrated above.

Hewstone, M., Stroebe, W., Codol, J.P., and Stephenson, G.M. (eds.) (1988) *Introduction to social psychology*. Blackwell, Oxford, p. 36.

3.5

   a **False.** Written by Thomas Szasz, a prominent 'anti-psychiatrist'.
   b **True.** Also 'clinical iatrogenesis' for the physical harm caused by medical intervention, and 'structural iatrogenesis' in which the medicalization of society undermines the individuals' autonomy and self-reliance.
   c **True.**
   d **True.**
   e **True.**

Patrick, D. and Scambler, G. (1982) *Sociology as applied to medicine.*. Ballière Tindall, London, pp. 176–81.

3.6

   a **False.** Thorndike—law of effect.
   b **True.** E.g. the presence of researchers enhancing the performance of subjects on various tests.
   c **False.** Wolpe—sytematic desensitization.
   d **False.** Bandura—social learning theory.
   e **True.**

Puri, B. and Tyrer, P. (1992) *Sciences basic to psychiatry*. Churchill Livingstone, Edinburgh, pp. 280–282, 288–289.

Questions

3.7   [Certainty]

With inborn errors of metabolism   High   Med   Low

   a Citrullinaemia is an example of an autosomal dominant   ...   .
urea cycle disorder.

   b Maple syrup urine disease will have a fatal outcome   ...   .
unless treated.

   c Effects of homocystinuria include skeletal abnormalities   ...   .
and rarely epilepsy.

   d Phenylketonuria (PKU) is the commonest inborn error of   ...   .
amino acid metabolism and leads to mental retardation.

   e A deficiency of tetrahydrobiopterin may cause PKU.   ...   .

3.8

The following conditions have a higher concordance rate in
monozygotic twins than in dizygotic twins:

   a Childhood autism.   ...   .

   b Anorexia nervosa.   ...   .

   c Panic disorder.   ...   .

   d Depressive disorder.   ...   .

   e Schizophrenia.   ...   .

3.9

Frontal release signs include

   a *Gegenhalten*.   ...   .

   b Palmomental reflex.   ...   .

   c Grasp reflex.   ...   .

   d Startle reflex.   ...   .

   e Encopresis.   ...   .

Answers

3.7

  a **False.** Autosomal recessive, as is the case for most inborn errors of metabolism.

  b **True.** Treatment includes a diet low in the three amino acids leucine, isoleucine, and valine.

  c **False.** Epilepsy is common.

  d **True.**

  e **True.** PKU is usually caused by deficiency of phenylalanine hydroxylase but can also be caused by tetrahydrobiopterin deficiency (the co-enzyme).

Puri, B. and Tyrer, P. (1992) *Sciences basic to psychiatry*. Churchill Livingstone, Edinburgh, pp. 77–79.

3.8

  a **True.**

  b **True.**

  c **True.**

  d **True.**

  e **True.**

Note: Studies in alcoholism have been conflicting. Twin studies on OCD have not been conclusive, although do suggest a genetic component.

Puri, B. and Tyrer, P. (1992) *Sciences basic to psychiatry*. Churchill Livingstone, Edinburgh, p. 166.

3.9

  a **False.** Counter-pull (or *gegenhalten*) is present when the patient actively resists attempts to passively flex or extend a limb joint. This is an indication of diffuse damage or degeneration, and is most often seen bilaterally.

  b **True.** Probably the most sensitive frontal release sign. Contraction of the mentalis muscle (between the lower lip and chin) after stimulating the thenar eminence (e.g. by drawing a key across it) indicates frontal cortical damage or degeneration on the opposite side.

  c **True.** A powerful grip on the fingers despite lifting away your hand is usually said to indicate severe frontal damage. Universal in infants up to 6 months.

  d **False.** Another primitive reflex. The limbs flex and the head and eyes orientate towards the startling stimulus. The reflex is mediated by the reticular formation via the superior and inferior colliculi, which are phylogenetically old relays.

  e **False.** Incontinence of faeces is seen at both ends of the life-cycle.

Morgan, G. and Butler, S. (eds.) (1993) *Seminars in basic neurosciences*. Gaskell, London, pp. 116–121.

Questions
3.10

[Certainty]

	High	Med	Low
Important factors determining normal ageing include			
a Errors in gene expression.	...	...	...
b Aluminium intake.	...	...	...
c Food restriction.	...	...	...
d Peroxidation rates.	...	...	...
e Declining availability of adenosine triphosphate (ATP).	...	...	...

3.11

The following deficits are the result of a right sided cerebral lesion:

a Acalculia.	...	...	...
b Anosognosia.	...	...	...
c Prosopagnosia.	...	...	...
d Gerstmann's syndrome.	...	...	...
e Constructional apraxia.	...	...	...

3.12

Regarding the neuropathology of schizophrenia:

a Brain weight and size are reduced.	...	...	...
b Gliotic reactions are often seen.	...	...	...
c A progressive loss of cerebral substance has been demonstrated.	...	...	...
d The hippocampus and anterior parahippocampal gyrus are particularly affected.	...	...	...
e The right temporal lobe is more affected than the left.	...	...	...

Answers

3.10

a **True.** Programmed ageing and somatic mutation, as well as epigenetic errors, are leading genetic theories behind ageing.

b **False.** Possibly has role in pathogenesis of some cases of Alzheimer's.

c **False.** Interestingly food restriction is associated with longevity.

d **True.** Oxidative damage by free radicals, generated as a by-product of respiration, could compromise the organism's ability to produce ATP and hence meet energy requirements.

e **True.** However, there is no evidence that antioxidants prolong life.

Jacoby, R and Oppenheimer, C. (1996) *Psychiatry in the elderly.* Oxford Medical Publications, Oxford, pp. 10–26.

3.11

a **False.** Dominant parietal lesions.

b **True.** A disorder of body image/failure to acknowledge illness on the opposite side of the body.

c **True.** Inability to recognize faces.

d **False.** Dominant parietal lesions.

e **True.**

Morgan, G and Butler, S. (eds.) (1993) *Seminars in basic neurosciences.* Gaskell, London, p. 30.

3.12

a **True.** A 2–6% decrease in brain weight, and approximately a 4% reduction in anterior–posterior length has been found in controlled studies. There is also some evidence that the normal asymmetries in the brain architecture are reduced or reversed.

b **False.** There is a paucity of neuronal gliotic reaction, which suggests that an early (perhaps migratory) deficit is involved rather than a later inflammatory reaction.

c **False.** Neuroimaging has revealed that any cerebral atrophy, or ventriculomegaly, is present at disease onset and is not progressive.

d **True.** Reduced cell number and abnormal cellular arrangement (pre-alpha cell migratory failure during 2nd trimester) are evident in the hippocampus and entorhinal cortex.

e **False.** The left appears consistently more affected than the right, particularly in the hippocampal region.

Note: This whole area of research was once described as a 'graveyard', and many findings seem contradictory or await replication. Perhaps the only other robust observation is of a comparative loss in cortical grey matter in schizophrenia.

Morgan, G and Butler, S. (eds.) (1993) *Seminars in basic neurosciences.* Gaskell, London, pp. 212–213.

Lawrie, S.M. and Abukmeil, S.S. (1998) Brain abnormality in schizophrenia. A systematic and quantitative review of volumetric magnetic resonance imaging studies. *British Journal of Psychiatry* 172, 110–120.

Questions
3.13

	[Certainty]		
The telencephalon develops into the	High	Med	Low
a Thalamus.	...	...	...
b Midbrain.	...	...	...
c Basal ganglia.	...	...	...
d Olfactory bulbs.	...	...	...
e Pons.	...	...	...

3.14

Concerning the spinal cord:

a The conus medullaris usually lies opposite the third or   ...   .
fourth lumbar vertebra by the age of 20.

b The posterior white columns are wholly occupied by   ...   .
ascending fibres.

c The anterior white columns contain pyramidal fibres and ...   .
vestibulospinal fibres.

d Cross sectional appearances of the spinal cord are similar ...   .
for the cervical, thoracic, and lumbar regions.

e Kinaesthetic sensation is relayed via the gracile and   ...   .
cuneate nuclei.

3.15

In drug metabolism and excretion

a Renal clearance decreases towards the end of pregnancy. ...   .

b Tricyclic antidepressants are present in breast milk in   ...   .
quantities too small to be harmful to the infant.

c Phenothiazines are relatively free from the effects of first- ...   .
pass metabolism.

d Monoamine oxidase is found only in brain and platelets. ...   .

e Opioid analgesics undergo hepatic biotransformation.   ...   .

Answers
3.13

a **False.** The thalamus is part of the diencephalon, a part of the forebrain that remains undivided in the midline.

b **False.** The midbrain, or mesencephalon, develops directly from the neural tube and changes very little remaining anchored to the centre of the cranial cavity.

c **True.** The telencephalon develops from the prosencephalon (forebrain) into the cerebral hemispheres and the basal ganglia.

d **True.** The olfactory bulbs and lobes comprise the rhinencephalon, arising out of the telencephalon.

e **False.** The pons, cerebellum and oral part of the medulla oblongata differentiate from the metencephalon, which in turn emerges from the rhombencephalon (hindbrain).

Kendell, R.E. and Zealley, A.K. (eds.) (1993) *Companion to psychiatric studies*, 5th edn. Churchill Livingstone, Edinburgh, pp. 82–83.

3.14

a **False.** Usually opposite the first or second lumbar vertebra.

b **True.** conveying light touch, moderate degrees of temperature variation and proprioception from joints, ligaments, tendons and muscles.

c **True.** Pyramidal fibres (from area 4 of the prefrontal gyrus), vestibulospinal (cell bodies in vestibular nucleus in the floor of the fourth ventricle).

d **False.** Cross sectional appearances of the spinal cord vary. The higher the level the greater the amount of grey matter.

e **True.** Kinaesthetic sensation is joint and muscle sense, spatial appreciation, and vibration sense.

McMinn, R.M.H. (1994) *Last's anatomy, regional and applied*, 9th edn. Churchill Livingstone, Edinburgh, pp. 619–626.

3.15

a **False.** Increases.

b **True.**

c **False.** There is great inter-individual variation. Up to 100% of the orally taken drug being metabolized by the liver on 'first-pass' in some individuals, hence the intramuscular route is better for some.

d **False.** Also found in liver, intestine, and kidney.

e **True.** Usually by oxidation in the smooth endoplasmic reticulum. They should be used with caution in liver disease.

Puri, B. and Tyrer, P. (1992) *Sciences basic to psychiatry*. Churchill Livingstone, Edinburgh, pp. 110–113.

Questions

3.16

	[Certainty]		
Serotonin (5HT)	High	Med	Low
a In the central nervous system accounts for less than 2% of the total body serotonin.	...	...	...
b Is synthesized from L-tryptophan.	...	...	...
c Storage is depleted by tetrabenazine.	...	...	...
d Release is dependent on sodium ions.	...	...	...
e Receptors of $5HT_{1A}$ subtype are located postsynaptically.	...	...	...

3.17

In development of new drugs the following phases of human trials are correctly described:

	High	Med	Low
a Phase II—Clinical investigations to confirm kinetics and dynamics in patients.	...	...	...
b Phase IV—Data analysis prior to marketing.	...	...	...
c Phase I—Pharmacological studies in animals.	...	...	...
d Phase V—Postmarketing surveillance to confirm safety of the drug.	...	...	...
e Phase III—Formal therapeutic trials in a large number of patients.	...	...	...

3.18

Therapeutic options contraindicated in pregnancy include

	High	Med	Low
a Electroconvulsive therapy (ECT).	...	...	...
b Carbamazepine.	...	...	...
c Phenelzine.	...	...	...
d Diazepam.	...	...	...
e Lithium carbonate.	...	...	...

Answers
3.16

a **True.** The rest is in intestine and platelets.

b **True.** By the action of tryptophan hydroxlase (the rate-limiting step).

c **True.** And also reserpine.

d **False.** Calcium.

e **True.** $5HT_{1A}$ receptors are also located presynaptically. Buspirone is a partial $5HT_{1A}$ agonist and has useful anti-anxiety effects.

Kendell, R.E. and Zealley, A.K. (eds.) (1993) *Companion to psychiatric studies*, 5th edn. Churchill Livingstone, Edinburgh, pp. 135–136.

3.17

a **True.**

b **False.** Phase IV is post-marketing surveillance.

c **False.** Phase I is studies of dynamics and kinetics in healthy volunteers.

d **False.** There is no Phase V.

e **True.**

Harry, J. (1991) Discovery and development of a new drug. *Prescriber's Journal* 31(6), 221–226.

3.18

a **False.** ECT is safe throughout pregnancy, although every anaesthetic carries a risk.

b **True.** Neural tube defects, craniofacial abnormalities, and a tendency to neonatal bleeding have been described.

c **False.** There is no evidence of harm, but manufacturers advise avoidance if possible.

d **False.** But neonatal floppiness and respiratory depression have been reported, along with a withdrawal syndrome. Shorter acting agents are thought to be preferred.

e **True.** This is controversial, but cardiac valve anomalies (particularly Ebstein's); neonatal goitre; and signs of toxicity in the neonate are seen. Current practice is to avoid in the first trimester particularly, although exposure to lithium is not an indication for abortion.

British National Formulary. Appendix 4 : Pregnancy.

Questions
3.19

<table>
<tr><td></td><td colspan="3">[Certainty]</td></tr>
<tr><td>Drugs leading to dependence include</td><td>High</td><td>Med</td><td>Low</td></tr>
<tr><td>a Triclofos sodium.</td><td>...</td><td>...</td><td>...</td></tr>
<tr><td>b Chlormethiazole.</td><td>...</td><td>...</td><td>...</td></tr>
<tr><td>c Meprobamate.</td><td>...</td><td>...</td><td>...</td></tr>
<tr><td>d Chlordiazepoxide.</td><td>...</td><td>...</td><td>...</td></tr>
<tr><td>e Zopiclone.</td><td>...</td><td>...</td><td>...</td></tr>
</table>

3.20

Physiological changes with ECT treatment include
a A decrease in blood–brain barrier permeability.
b A rise in plasma cortisol.
c A fall in plasma ACTH and GH levels.
d Vagal stimulation of the heart.
e A rise in plasma prolactin levels.

3.21

The following statements are true:
a Pain acts as a stimulus for antidiuretic hormone (ADH) release.
b Chronic alcohol ingestion has been shown to increase ADH levels in plasma.
c Research findings have shown a general suprahypothalamic underactivity in depression.
d Cholecystokinin (CCK) is found in high concentrations in the limbic system.
e Classical and operant conditioning has been shown to be affected by corticotrophin and vasopressin related peptides.

3.22

During sleep
a In normal males, rapid eye movement (REM) is invariably associated with penile erections.
b In depressive illness, there is no effect on penile erections during REM.
c REM latency has been shown to increase in depression.
d The total amount of REM sleep is decreased in depression.
e A positive response to treatment in depression may be predicted by prompt change in REM latency on starting antidepressants.

Answers

3.19

a **True.** A derivative of chloral hydrate which is said to cause fewer gastro-intestinal side-effects.

b **True.** Intended as a hypnotic only in the elderly and very short-term use in assisted withdrawal from alcohol in younger adults.

c **True.** Less effective than benzodiazepines and more hazardous in overdose.

d **True.** A long-acting benzodiazepine used to attenuate alcohol withdrawal symptoms.

e **False.** This is somewhat controversial, as it is still a relatively new product. Again only for short-term use.

British National Formulary. Section 4.1.

3.20

a **False.** There is an increase in permeability and cerebral blood flow.

b **True.** This lasts for approximately 2–4 hours.

c **False.** These substances rise in concentration.

d **True.** This slowing can be countered by administering atropine, 'vagal blockade'.

e **True.** This test can also help distinguish between seizures and pseudoseizures.

3.21

a **True.** Emotional stress and pain stimulate ADH and ACTH release.

a **True.**

c **False.** Overactivity.

d **True.** As well as cerebral cortex.

e **True.**

Puri, B. and Tyrer, P. (1992) *Sciences basic to psychiatry*. Churchill Livingstone, Edinburgh, pp. 42–46.

3.22

a **True.** Important in differentiating organic and psychogenic causes of impotence.

b **False.** There may be a failure of this in depressed patients.

c **False.** It decreases.

d **False.** It is increased, especially in the first third of the night.

e **True.**

Kendell, R.E. and Zealley, A.K. (eds.) (1993) *Companion to psychiatric studies*, 5th edn. Churchill Livingstone, Edinburgh, pp. 543–547.

Questions
3.23

[Certainty]

According to Kohlberg's theories of moral development	High	Med	Low
a There are four levels of morality.	...	...	...
b Stages are parallel to those of Piaget's stages of cognitive development.	...	...	...
c Often children do not progress through stages sequentially.	...	...	...
d The highest stages are very rarely achieved and cannot be regarded as normal.	...	...	...
e Only 50% of the population reach the highest level of moral development (ethical principle orientation).	...	...	...

3.24

'Learned helplessness' research

a Is based on classic work by Beck.	...	...	...
b Shows that animals learn by observing the futile efforts of others.	...	...	...
c Was originally carried out on rats.	...	...	...
d Gives an explanation for psychomotor retardation in depressed people.	...	...	...
e Suggests that depressive illness should be dichotomized into endogenous and reactive subtypes.	...	...	...

3.25

In the assessment of personality

a Extroverted behaviour has been suggested as being due to excessive cortical arousal.	...	...	...
b Skin conductance has been shown to differ between introverts and extroverts.	...	...	...
c 'Irrational ' and 'moody' are two traits on the psychoticism spectrum according to Eysenck.	...	...	...
d Graphology has been shown to be a useful technique for personality disorder assessment.	...	...	...
e Both the Rorschach and the thematic apperception tests are examples of projective tests.	...	...	...

Answers
3.23

    a **False.** There are 3 levels—pre-conventional, conventional, and post-conventional.

    b **True.**

    c **False.** The development of moral thinking proceeds through sequential steps.

    d **True.**

    e **False.** Less than 10%.

Black, D. and Cottrell, D. (eds.) (1993) *Seminars in child and adolescent psychiatry*. Gaskell, London, pp. 23–24.

3.24

    a **False.** Seligman.

    b **False.** It shows that animals given aversive stimuli from which they are unable to escape become passive, and later do not attempt to escape even when able to do so.

    c **False.** This research was carried out in the laboratory using dogs.

    d **True.** Similar features are seen in animals and depressed humans, i.e. reduced voluntary movements and a resignation that one has no control over the environment.

    e **False.**

Puri, B. and Tyrer, P. (1992) *Sciences basic to psychiatry*. Churchill Livingstone, Edinburgh, pp. 282.

3.25

    a **False.** Habitual low cortical arousal.

    b **True.** As a measure of arousal. Found to be higher in introverts.

    c **False.** Neuroticism.

    d **False.** Analysis of handwriting—there is little evidence for validity.

    e **True.** Although they have low validity.

Tantum, D. and Birchwood, M. (eds.) (1994) *Seminars in psychology and the social sciences*. Gaskell, London. pp. 187–200.

Questions

Clinical

3.26

[Certainty]

Concerning depressive illness in the elderly:

	High	Med	Low
a The short term prognosis is good.	...	...	...
b About 10% are resistant to all conventional therapies.	...	...	...
c Patients are rarely seriously suicidal.	...	...	...
d It is present in about 15% of the elderly population.	...	...	...
e A cardiac pacemaker is an absolute contraindication to ECT.	...	...	...

3.27

The following abnormalities have been described in depression:

	High	Med	Low
a Reduced ventricular to brain ratios.	...	...	...
b Hypofrontality on positron emission tomography (PET).	...	...	...
c Abnormal eye-tracking movements.	...	...	...
d Abnormal P300 event-related potential amplitudes.	...	...	...
e A prolonged interval between the onset of sleep and the first period of rapid eye movement sleep (REM).	...	...	...

3.28

The following features help establish a diagnosis of schizoaffective disorder rather than any other disorder:

	High	Med	Low
a Schizophrenia in a first degree relative.	...	...	...
b Continuing low mood after resolution of a psychotic episode.	...	...	...
c Mood-incongruent hallucinations during a severe depressive episode.	...	...	...
d Episodic but chronic course.	...	...	...
e Simultaneous prominent schizophrenic and affective symptoms.	...	...	...

Answers

Clinical

3.26

a **True.** But the long-term prognosis is not favourable for at least 40% of cases.

b **True.** Up to one third of cases are left with disabling symptoms.

c **False.** The elderly account for 25% of all suicides, but a mere 5% of recorded attempts.

d **False.** Depressive illness is seen in about 3%, whereas depressive symptoms are present in 10–15% of the community.

e **False.** The patient should be totally insulated, and not touched during the electrical impulse.

Jacoby, R. and Oppenheimer, C. (eds.) (1991) *Psychiatry in the elderly.* Oxford Medical Publications, Oxford, pp. 676–720.

3.27

a **False.** Increased ventricular to brain ratios have been well described in depression and schizophrenia using a variety of neuroimaging techniques.

b **True.** Reduced perfusion seen in frontotemporal regions has been shown in some studies to reverse with clinical recovery.

c **True.** This has also been described in schizophrenia.

d **True.** This has also been described in schizophrenia.

e **False.** A shortened interval (reduced REM latency) is described in depressive disorder.

Kendell, R.E. and Zealley, A.K. (eds.) (1993).*Companion to psychiatric studies,* 5th edn. Churchill Livingstone, Edinburgh, pp. 427–453.

3.28

a **False.** Several studies do suggest an increased risk of schizophrenia in first-degree relatives for schizoaffective disorder, but this does not differentiate from schizophrenia itself.

b **False.** This is common after any psychotic episode.

c **False.** Does not by itself justify a diagnosis of schizoaffective disorder over an affective disorder.

d **False.** This is characteristic of schizoaffective disorder but also of a severe bipolar affective disorder.

e **True.** These two categories of symptom must be definite and prominent, and occur simultaneously or within a few days of each other.

World Health Organization (1992). *Tenth revision of the International Classification of Disease (ICD 10).* WHO, Geneva, pp. 105–8.

Questions

3.29

[Certainty]

During the puerperium

	High	Med	Low

a Around 5% of mothers become clinically depressed within 6 weeks of childbirth.

b Breast-feeding may be continued during treatment with tricyclic antidepressants.

c The risk of developing a postpartum psychosis is higher in primagravidae.

d Psychosis is more likely to be schizophrenic than manic.

e Those at risk of a puerperal psychosis have been shown to have increased dopamine receptor sensitivity in the hypothalamus.

3.30

Laboratory investigations commonly found to be abnormal in anorexia nervosa include:

a Hypercarotenaemia.

b Lowered plasma cortisol.

c Leukocytosis.

d Hyperuricaemia.

e Raised plasma amylase.

3.31

The following help define a phobia:

a Autonomic symptoms which are secondary to obsessional or delusional thoughts.

b Avoidance of the feared stimuli and any treatment using the feared stimuli.

c An anticipatory fear that cannot be explained or reasoned away.

d Anxiety that is helped by others not viewing the feared stimuli as dangerous or threatening.

e Fear that is beyond voluntary control.

Answers
3.29

   a **False.** 15–20% of mothers.

   b **True.** The amount of tricyclics excreted is too small to be harmful but along with SSRIs most manufacturers advise avoidance. Lithium should be avoided if possible. If lithium is necessary, it is advised to monitor the infant for toxicity and closely monitor maternal lithium levels.

   c **True.**

   d **False.** Affective presentations are more common than schizophrenic or organic types.

   e **True.**

British National Formulary, Appendix 5.

Gelder, M., Gath, D., Mayou, R., and Cowen, P. (eds.) (1996) *The Oxford textbook of psychiatry*, 3rd edn. Oxford University Press, Oxford, pp. 395–397.

Kendell, R.E. and Zealley, A.K. (eds.) (1993) *Companion to psychiatric studies*, 5th edn. Churchill Livingstone, Edinburgh, pp. 579–582.

3.30

   a **True.**

   b **False.** Cortisol levels are raised.

   c **False.** Usually a leucopaenia with a relative lymphocytosis.

   d **False.** Low uric acid levels.

   e **True.**

Freeman, C.P.L. and Sharp, C.W. (1993) The medical complications of anorexia nervosa. *British Journal of Psychiatry* 162, 452–462.

3.31

   a **False.** The psychological and autonomic symptoms are primary manifestations of anxiety, and not secondary to delusions or obsessions.

   b **False.** There is avoidance of the feared stimuli, but not of carefully constructed desensitisation techniques.

   c **True.**

   d **False.** The anxiety is not relieved by the knowledge that others do not view the situation as dangerous or threatening.

   e **True.**

World Health Organization (1992) *Tenth revision of the International Classification of Disease (ICD 10)*. WHO, Geneva, pp. 134–8.

Questions
3.32
[Certainty]

Disulfiram   High Med Low
  a Exerts its action by inhibiting alcohol dehydrogenase.   ...   .
  b Reduces the levels of concurrently administered phenytoin.   ...   .
  c Should be given as a loading dose when commencing use as a deterrent for alcohol dependence.   ...   .
  d Alcohol reactions persist for up to 3 days.   ...   .
  e Is contraindicated in patients with elevated liver enzymes.   ...   .

3.33
The following drugs have been reported as being effective in patients with borderline personality disorder:
  a High-dose neuroleptics.   ...   .
  b Low-dose neuroleptics.   ...   .
  c Monoamine oxidase inhibitors.   ...   .
  d Lithium.   ...   .
  e Carbamazepine.   ...   .

3.34
Pimozide
  a Is more sedating than chlorpromazine.   ...   .
  b Is safe in breast-feeding.   ...   .
  c Treatment should be preceded by an electrocardiogram (ECG) in all patients.   ...   .
  d Treatment should incorporate annual ECGs in patients who are maintained on doses over 16 mg per day.   ...   .
  e Can be given safely with other antipsychotics.   ...   .

Answers
3.32

a **False.** Exerts its action by inhibiting acetaldehyde dehydrogenase, leading to raised levels of acetaldehyde which are responsible for the unpleasant 'antabuse' reaction: nausea, flushing, headache, palpitations, dizziness, and sometimes dyspnoea.

b **False.** Disulfiram is an enzyme inhibitor and will therefore increase levels of phenytoin, barbiturates, diazepam, warfarin, pethidine, theophyllines, and metronidazole.

c **True.** E.g. day 1–800 mg; day 2–600 mg; day 3–400 mg; thereafter 200 mg daily.

d **False.** Seven days, and patients should be warned about this.

e **False.** Disulfiram is contraindicated in patients with advanced liver disease, i.e. serum bilirubin >25 mmol l^{-1} and low serum albumin. Elevated enzymes, i.e. gamma GT and transaminases, occur in two thirds of patients with alcohol problems and gamma GT levels improve with adherence to disulfiram therapy (because they drink less).

Chick, J. (1996) Medication in the treatment of alcohol dependence. *Advances in Psychiatric Treatment* 2, 249–257.

Cookson, J., Crammer, J. and Heine, B. (1993) *The use of drugs in psychiatry*, 3rd edn. Gaskell, London, pp. 298–299.

3.33

a **False.**
b **True.**
c **True.**
d **False.**
e **True.**

Stein, G. and Wilkinson, G. (eds.) (1998) *Seminars in general adult psychiatry*, Vol. 2. Gaskell, London, pp. 841–852.

3.34

a **False.** It is less sedating than other antipsychotics, e.g. chlorpromazine.

b **False.** It is contra-indicated in breast-feeding.

c **True.** The Committee on Safety on Medicines (CSM) recommend not giving pimozide with drugs which may prolong the QT interval on the ECG, e.g. anti-arrhythmics, antimalarials and antihistamines, and drugs that may cause electrolyte disturbance such as diuretics.

d **True.**

e **False.** The CSM recommends that pimozide should not be given with any other antipsychotics including depot preparations.

British National Formulary, Section 4.2.

Questions
3.35   [Certainty]

	High	Med	Low
In the treatment of schizophrenia			
a Tardive dyskinesia does not occur in patients who have never been treated with antipsychotics.	...	...	...
b The atypical antipsychotic clozapine is thought to block dopamine D_2 receptors.	...	...	...
c Clozapine should be prescribed to those patients who present with predominantly negative symptoms.	...	...	...
d Butyrephenones are more likely to cause extrapyramidal side effects than phenothiazines.	...	...	...
e To prevent extrapyramidal side-effects, it is good practice to prescribe regular procyclidine as a matter of routine with thioridazine.	...	...	...

3.36

Regarding delirium tremens:

	High	Med	Low
a There is a mortality of 25–30%.	...	...	...
b Fear is a characteristic symptom.	...	...	...
c Vitamin B_{12} should be given routinely.	...	...	...
d It may occur in those not physically dependent on alcohol.	...	...	...
e Nitrous oxide can be a helpful treatment.	...	...	...

3.37

Migraine:

	High	Med	Low
a Affects 0.5—1% of the population at one time or another.	...	...	...
b Rarely has an onset before the age of 10.	...	...	...
c Symptoms may be temporarily relieved by pregnancy.	...	...	...
d Of the basilar artery may cause alterations of consciousness.	...	...	...
e Can be usefully treated by using biofeedback techniques.	...	...	...

Answers
3.35
  a **False.** Tardive dyskinesia occurs in drug naive patients.
  b **True.** Amongst other receptors.
  c **False.** Clozapine should be reserved for those patients who have not responded to adequate trials of at least two conventional antipsychotics, or those intolerant of conventional agents.
  d **True.** Butyrephenones are more likely to cause extrapyramidal side effects than phenothiazines.
  e **False.** Routine prescription of anticholinergics with antipsychotics should be avoided as this may contribute to development of tardive dyskinesia. In addition thioridazine is an antipsychotic with marked anticholinergic effects in its own right.

Cookson, J., Crammer, J. and Heine, B. (1993) *The use of drugs in psychiatry*, 3rd edn. Gaskell, London, pp. 233–262, 298–299,

Kendell, R.E. and Zealley, A.K. (eds.) (1993) *Companion to psychiatric studies,* 5th edn. Churchill Livingstone, Edinburgh, pp. 397–423.

3.36
  a **False.** This used to be the case, but mortality is now under 15%. Nevertheless, the gravity of delirium tremens can be overlooked.
  b **True.** Also agitation, sleeplessness (with REM sleep rebound), and autonomic overactivity are often seen.
  c **False.** Thiamine (B_1) is the treatment for Wernicke's encephalopathy. However, parenteral vitamins B and C (Pabrinex) are often given in delirium tremens.
  d **False.**
  e **True.** The analgesic nitrous oxide has been used to abolish alcohol withdrawal symptoms. Other less common treatments include clonidine, dexamethasone, and alcohol.

Chick, J. and Cantwell, R. (eds.) (1994) *Seminars in alcohol and drug misuse.* Gaskell, London, pp. 133–4, 174–6.

3.37
  a **False.** It is much commoner, 5–10%.
  b **False.** The onset is before the age of 10 in 25% of cases and often presents with abdominal symptoms, e.g. episodic abdominal pain.
  c **True.**
  d **True.** The basilar artery is formed by the two vertebral arteries and supplies the brain stem.
  e **True.**

Lishman, W.A. (1998) *Organic psychiatry*, 3rd edn. Blackwell Science, Oxford, pp. 399–410.

Questions
3.38

	[Certainty]		
The following statements are true:	High	Med	Low
a Psychogenic polydipsia is an occasional symptom of schizophrenia.	...	...	...
b Hyperthermia may be a symptom in Korsakoff's syndrome.	...	...	...
c Lesions in Korsakoff's syndrome and Wernicke's encephalopathy are similar.	...	...	...
d Pick's disease has equal sex incidence.	...	...	...
e Glycosuria is a feature of Wilson's disease.	...	...	...

3.39

In syphilitic infections of the brain the following are seen in more than 50% of cases:

a Argyll Robertson pupil.	...	...	...
b Tremor of the limbs.	...	...	...
c Dysarthria.	...	...	...
d Tabes dorsalis.	...	...	...
e Depressive illness.	...	...	...

3.40

The Kleine–Levin syndrome

a Is due to diencephalic dysfunction.	...	...	...
b Is characterized by periodic insomnia.	...	...	...
c Usually affects young females.	...	...	...
d Has megaphagia as a symptom.	...	...	...
e Is associated with hypersexuality.	...	...	...

Answers

3.38

a **True.** This is characterized by excessive water intake and can result in significant hyponatraemia, leading to convulsions, coma, and death.

b **False.** Hypothermia may be seen.

c **True.** Both are cerebral consequences of vitamin B_1 deficiency and manifest as petechial haemorrhages in the mammillary bodies and periventricular areas.

d **False.** Females are affected twice as often as males, in this frontotemporal dementia.

e **True.** Renal copper deposition may cause aminoaciduria, glycosuria, proteinuria, and decreased glomerular filtration rate. Renal presentations of Wilson's disease are rare; hepatic and neurological presentations are more usual.

Puri, B. and Tyrer P. (1992).*Sciences basic to psychiatry*. Churchill Livingstone, Edinburgh, pp. 181–197.

3.39

a **True.** Argyll Robertson pupil is present in approximately two-thirds of patients.

b **True.** As well as the tongue.

c **True.** Dysarthria is said to be present in 80%.

d **False.** 20% have tabes dorsalis (spinal cord involvement).

e **False.** Depressive illness is present in approximately 27% according to one series.

Lishman, W.A. (1998) *Organic psychiatry*, 3rd edn. Blackwell Science, Oxford, pp. 338–341.

3.40

a **True.** Probably a hypothalamic disorder, as both the appetite and sleep–wake cycle are disturbed.

b **False.** The periodic hypersomnia occurs in bouts lasting a few days to a few weeks, with normality in between. If the sufferer is roused (with difficulty) from sleep they can be irritable.

c **False.** It is a rare disorder affecting young males. Lithium can be a useful treatment.

d **True.** Excessive appetite is also known as hyperphagia. Straightforward obesity and atypical bulimia should be excluded.

e **True.**

Lishman, W.A. (1998) *Organic psychiatry*, 3rd edn. Blackwell Science, Oxford, pp. 732–733.

Questions
3.41

[Certainty]

The following are associated with a low incidence of alcoholism:

	High	Med	Low
a Alcoholic beverages considered mainly as a food and usually consumed with meals.	...	...	...
b Exposure to alcohol as a child, early in life, in the context of a strong family or religious group.	...	...	...
c Parents presenting a constant example of moderate drinking.	...	...	...
d Ship's deckhands and navigators.	...	...	...
e A culture of complete abstinence.	...	...	...

3.42

In the treatment of opiate addiction

a Dilatation of the pupils may be a sign of opiate withdrawal.	...	...	...
b Only specially registered practitioners may prescribe methadone.	...	...	...
c All suspected addicts must be notified to the local Health Authority.	...	...	...
d Co-phenotrope is useful in alleviating withdrawal symptoms.	...	...	...
e β-Adrenoceptor blockade is useful in alleviating withdrawal symptoms.	...	...	...

3.43

With regard to psychiatry and the law:

a Infanticide is defined as the killing of a child under 1 month by the mother or father.	...	...	...
b Exhibitionism is a form of paraphilia.	...	...	...
c The majority of indecent exposers will go on to commit more serious sexual offences.	...	...	...
d Patients with schizophrenia show increased rates of offending compared to the general public.	...	...	...
e The inability of a patient to instruct his or her lawyer would prevent him or her being deemed fit to plead.	...	...	...

Answers
3.41

a **True.** a, b, and c are based on a review of childhood and adolescent drinking behaviour. Other factors include intoxication being socially unacceptable and drinking not being perceived as adult or virile.

b **True.**

c **True.**

d **False.** After publicans, seamen are amongst the most likely occupational group to die from liver cirrhosis.

e **False.** There is evidence from Islamic culture and American prohibition that this is ineffective, if not counterproductive.

Chick, J and Cantwell, R. (eds.) (1994) *Seminars in alcohol and drug misuse.* Gaskell, London, pp. 113–115.

3.42

a **True.**

b **False.** Any doctor may prescribe methadone.

c **False.** Addicts must be notified to the Chief Medical Officer.

d **True.** This drug helps reduce gut motility; it is marketed as Lomotil.

e **True.** E.g. propranolol may provide some symptomatic relief by reducing anxiety symptoms.

Gerada, C. and Ashworth, M. (1997) Addiction and dependence—I: illicit drugs. *British Medical Journal* 315, 297–300.

3.43

a **False.** This is the killing of a child under 1 year by the mother.

b **True.**

c **False.** Less than 20% re-offend.

d **False.** Patients with schizophrenia show a similar rate of offending as the general public.

e **True.** Being fit to plead include being able to understand the nature of the charge and the proceedings of the court, and abilities to instruct a lawyer (counsel) and challenge a juror.

Chiswick, D. and Cope R. (eds.) (1995) *Seminars in forensic psychiatry.* Gaskell, London, pp. 40, 110, 119.

Questions
3.44   [Certainty]

The following increase the risk of a psychiatric patient causing   High   Med   Low
harm to another:

    a Previous suicidal behaviour.   ...   .
    b Recent discontinuation of medication.   ...   .
    c Persecutory delusions.   ...   .
    d Childhood abuse.   ...   .
    e Thought withdrawal.   ...   .

3.45

Depression in middle childhood

    a Is more common in girls than boys.   ...   .
    b May be assessed using the 'Kiddie-SADS'.   ...   .
    c Usually presents with 'vegetative' symptoms.   ...   .
    d Is usually treated with pharmacotherapy.   ...   .
    e Is less common than in early adolescence.   ...   .

3.46

The following are true of learning difficulty:

    a The prevalence of learning difficulty decreases with age   ...   .
       until the late teenage years.
    b The prevalence of moderate and severe handicap has been ...   .
       found to be reasonably constant at 9 per 1000.
    c Rhesus incompatibility is a recognized cause of learning   ...   .
       difficulty.
    d The majority of cerebral palsy sufferers have IQs in the   ...   .
       mentally handicapped range.
    e About 5% of all foetuses have chromosomal abnormalities. ...   .

3.47

Sigmund Freud

    a Was born in Vienna.   ...   .
    b Was an habitual user of cocaine.   ...   .
    c Wrote *Studies on hysteria* with Wilhelm Fleiss.   ...   .
    d Wrote *The interpretation of dreams*.   ...   .
    e Died in New York.   ...   .

Answers
3.44

a **True.** As well as previous violence.

b **True.** Poor compliance and recent losses heighten risk.

c **True.** Phenomena of threat or control (e.g. passivity) increase risk.

d **False.** Poor social stability and substance misuse are worrying background factors.

e **False.**

Royal College of Psychiatrists' Council Report CR 53. (April 1996) *Assessment and clinical management of risk of harm to other people.* RCPsych, London.

3.45

a **False.** It is more common in boys.

b **True.** This is a semistructured interview for children and adolescents.

c **False.** More usually sadness, helplessness, loneliness, boredom, social withdrawal, etc.

d **False.** Other treatments such as individual, cognitive, or family therapy are more usual.

e **True.** Mood disorders become much more common in adolescence.

Black, D. and Cottrell, D. (eds.) (1993) *Seminars in child and adolescent psychiatry.* Gaskell, London, pp. 128–129.

3.46

a **False.** Learning difficulty increases with age until the late teens and thereafter declines.

b **False.** 3.7 per 1000.

c **True.**

d **False.** Around 50% have normal or above normal intelligence.

e **True.** About 90% of these abort.

Kendell, R.E. and Zealley, A.K. (eds.) (1993) *Companion to psychiatric studies,* 5th edn. Churchill Livingstone, Edinburgh, pp. 623–629.

3.47

a **False.** Freiberg, Moravia.

b **True.**

c **False.** This was co-authored with Josef Breuer.

d **True.**

e **False.** Freud died in London in 1939.

Jacobs, M. (1992) *Sigmund Freud* (Key Figures in Counselling and Psychotherapy Series). Sage, London.

Questions
3.48

	[Certainty]		
Supportive psychotherapy differs from explorative psychotherapy in that	High	Med	Low
a The subject's defences are confronted.	...	...	...
b Advice is given.	...	...	...
c Medication is offered.	...	...	...
d The subject is allowed to regress.	...	...	...
e The subject is allowed to ventilate his/her feelings.	...	...	...

3.49

In brief dynamic psychotherapy

	High	Med	Low
a Treatment lasts less than 20 sessions.	...	...	...
b The therapist is more active than in longer term therapy.	...	...	...
c Efforts are made to find a focus early in treatment.	...	...	...
d Patients with personality disorders are excluded from treatment.	...	...	...
e Issues to do with termination are addressed early in treatment.	...	...	...

3.50

The following culture-bound disorders are correctly paired with their characteristic clinical features

	High	Med	Low
a Dhat—Fear of penis retracting into abdomen.	...	...	...
b Susto—Delusions that the subject has turned into a cannibalistic monster.	...	...	...
c Windigo—Anxiety regarding loss of one's soul.	...	...	...
d Latah—Depressive withdrawal followed by an indiscriminate murderous frenzy.	...	...	...
e Amok—Semen loss or erectile dysfunction.	...	...	...

Answers
3.48

    a **False.** The subject's defences are supported and reinforced in supportive therapy whereas they are often confronted and modified in explorative therapy.

    b **True.** But withheld in explorative therapy.

    c **True.** Medication is discouraged in explorative therapy.

    d **False.** The subject is allowed to regress (within sessions) in explorative therapy.

    e **False.** This is acceptable in both forms of therapy.

Brown, D. and Pedder, J. (1991) *Introduction to psychotherapy*, 2nd edn. Routledge, London, p. 100.

3.49

    a **False.** Therapy may last up to 40 sessions

    b **True.**

    c **True.**

    d **False.**

    e **True.**

Holmes, J. (1994) Brief dynamic psychotherapy. *Advances in Psychiatric Treatment* 1, 9–15.

3.50

    a **False.** Dhat—A psychosexual disorder found in Asian countries characterized by fear of semen loss or erectile dysfunction.

    b **False.** Susto—An acute anxiety state regarding the loss of one's sole, or social role.

    c **False.** Windigo—Thought to be a variant of depressive psychosis with accompanying delusions that the subject has turned into a cannibalistic monster.

    d **False.** Latah—A dissociative state with echolalia and automatic obedience. Found in the Far East and North Africa.

    e **False.** Amok—Possibly a depressive or dissociative state characterized by a period of withdrawal, followed by an indiscriminate murderous frenzy.

Note: Koro is an acute anxiety disorder related to the fear of the penis retracting into the abdomen. It is found in south-east Asian countries.

Buckey P. F., Bird, J. and Harrison, G. (1995) *Examination notes in psychiatry*, 3rd edn. Butterworth-Heinemann, Oxford, p. 387.

Paper 4: Questions

Basic science

4.1

With regard to measures of reliability and validity:

	High	Med	Low
	[Certainty]		

a The weighted kappa statistic (κ_w) allows for chance agreement in measuring agreement between observers. ... ...

b Concurrent validity is synonymous with face validity. ... ...

c Predictive validity is relatively straightforward to measure. ... ...

d Concurrent validity is used to indicate whether one measure is superior to another in approaching true validity. ... ...

e Concurrent and predictive validity together are sometimes known as criterion validity. ... ...

4.2

Regarding the lod score:

a It is the common log of the odds ratio. ... ...

b It is a method of assessing the likelihood of genetic linkage. ... ...

c Conventionally a value of 3 or over is taken to exclude linkage. ... ...

d Any multiple testing should be corrected for before interpreting the lod score. ... ...

e It is derived from the recombination fraction produced by meiosis. ... ...

4.3

Rating scales are commonly used in psychiatric research.

a The Hamilton Depression Rating Scale (HDRS) can be used as a diagnostic instrument. ... ...

b The Beck Depression Inventory (BDI) is a self-rating scale. ... ...

c The Montgomery and Asperg Depression Rating Scale (MADRS) is sensitive to change. ... ...

d The Brief Psychiatric Rating Scale (BPRS) is a purely observer based rating scale. ... ...

e The General Health Questionnaire (GHQ) was designed to be used in community settings. ... ...

Paper 4: Answers

Basic science

4.1

a **True.** Therefore sometimes more appropriate than the product–moment correlation coefficient for measuring inter-rater reliability.

b **False.** Concurrent validity describes whether the measure being tested is true by the use of an independent, validated measure. Face validity is a subjective assessment of whether a measure appears to be measuring what it is supposed to be.

c **False.** Whether something measured in the present (e.g. alcohol abuse) will predict future events (e.g. suicide).

d **False.** This is known as incremental validity.

e **True.**

Puri, B. and Tyrer, P. (1992) *Sciences basic to psychiatry*. Churchill Livingstone, Edinburgh, pp. 256–258.

4.2

a **False.** Lod is 'log of the odds'. It is the common log of the likelihood that the recombination fraction has a certain value.

b **True.** Answer suggested by part c.

c **False.** A lod score of at least 3 represents an odds of linkage of 1000 : 1, and is the accepted level for concluding linkage has been detected (95% reliability). A lod score of –2 excludes linkage.

d **True.** Multiple testing can artificially lead to significance in many areas, giving false positives.

e **True.** The recombination fraction is the number of recombinants (i.e. crossed-over offspring during meiosis) divided by the total number of offspring.

McGuffin, P., Owen, M. J., O'Donovan, M.C., Thapar, A., and Gottesman, I.I. (1994) *Seminars in psychiatric genetics*. Gaskell, London, pp. 55–58.

4.3

a **False.** The HDRS should only be used on those who have already been diagnosed and used specifically to rate severity of depression.

b **True.**

c **True.** It is more useful than the HDRS when assessing people with concurrent physical illness because it is more concerned with psychological rather than the physical symptoms of depression.

d **False.** 11 items are by verbal report, 5 are observed behaviour.

e **True.**

Kendell, R.E. and Zealley, A.K. (eds.) (1993) *Companion to psychiatric studies*, 5th edn. Churchill Livingstone, Edinburgh, pp. 172–175.

Questions

4.4

[Certainty]

In the evaluation of diagnostic instruments

	High	Med	Low

a The sensitivity of a test is the (number of true positives)   ...   .
divided by (the number of true positives plus the number
of false positives).

b The specificity of a test is (the number of true negatives)   ...   .
divided by (the number of true negatives plus the
number of false positives).

c The predictive value of a positive test result is the   ...   .
proportion of positive test results that are truly positive.

d The efficiency of a test is the proportion of all results   ...   .
that is true.

e The validity of a test is (the number of true positives plus   ...   .
true negatives) minus (the number of false negatives plus
false positives).

4.5

The following neuroanatomical statements are true.

a The internal carotid arteries give rise to corresponding   ...   .
anterior cerebral arteries.

b Tumours of the pituitary gland can present with   ...   .
bitemporal hemianopia.

c The inferior aspects of the temporal lobes are supplied by   ...   .
the middle cerebral artery.

d The anterior spinal artery is formed from branches of the   ...   .
posterior cerebral arteries.

e With regard to the motor cortex (prefrontal gyrus), ...
pyramidal cells innervating the upper limb lie more
medially than cells innervating the lower limb.

4.6

Correct statements regarding brain structure and function
include the following:

a The rhinencephalon is derived from the telencephalon.   ...   .

b The corpus striatum consists of claustrum and   ...   .
amygdaloid nucleus.

c The superior colliculi are involved primarily with   ...   .
auditory reflexes.

d The thalamus forms the lateral wall of the fourth   ...   .
ventricle.

e The pineal gland forms part of the epithalamus.   ...   .

Answers
4.4

    a **False.** True positives divided by true positives plus false negatives.
    b **True.**
    c **True.**
    d **True.**
    e **False.** Validity of a test is measured by different criteria.

Note: The best diagnostic tests have high sensitivity (to detect cases) and high specificity (to avoid including non-cases)

Puri, B. and Tyrer, P. (1992) *Sciences basic to psychiatry*. Churchill Livingstone, Edinburgh, pp. 273–274.

4.5

    a **True.**
    b **True.** The pituitary gland is in close proximity to the optic chiasm. Depending on the direction of the tumour growth a variety of visual defects are described including the one stated.
    c **False.** The inferior aspects of the temporal lobes are supplied by the posterior cerebral artery.
    d **False.** The anterior spinal artery is formed from union of the two vertebral arteries.
    e **False.** This is best worked out by noting the motor homunculus. Cells innervating the upper limb lie more laterally than cells innervating the lower limb.

McMinn, R.M.H. (1994) *Last's anatomy, regional and applied*, 9th edn. Churchill Livingstone, Edinburgh, pp. 600–605.

4.6

    a **True.** Telencephalion gives rise to cortex rhinencephalon, corpus striatum, and medullary centre.
    b **False.** These are components of the basal ganglia but not strictly part of the corpus striatum which consists of the caudate and lentiform nuclei.
    c **False.** They are involved in visual reflexes.
    d **False.** Lateral wall of the third ventricle.
    e **True.** Also the habenular nuclei.

Puri, B. and Tyrer, P. (1992) *Sciences basic to psychiatry*. Churchill Livingstone, Edinburgh, pp. 6–9.

Questions
4.7
[Certainty]

Characteristic neuropathological features of the 'punch-drunk' High Med Low
syndrome include

    a A fenestrated septum pellucidum.   ... ...

    b Degeneration of the substantia nigra.   ... ...

    c Neuronal loss in the cerebral cortex and the cerebellum. ... ...

    d Cortical neurofibrillary tangle formation similar to   ... ...
Alzheimer's disease.

    e Diffuse cortical β-amyloid plaques.   ... ...

4.8

Brain regions implicated in the Wernicke–Korsakoff syndrome
include

    a Paraventricular parts of the thalamus.   ... ...

    b Paraventricular parts of the hypothalamus.   ... ...

    c Mammillary bodies.   ... ...

    d Periaqueductal grey matter of the midbrain.   ... ...

    e Floor of the fourth ventricle.   ... ...

4.9

Neurocellular reactions to disease include:

    a Hirano bodies, occurring rarely in Alzheimer's disease.   ... ...

    b Pick bodies, consisting of neurofilaments, paired helical ... ...
filaments and endoplasmic reticulum.

    c Lewy bodies, mainly found in neocortex.   ... ...

    d Neurofibrillary tangles, in patients with postencephalitic ... ...
parkinsonism.

    e Granulovacuolar degeneration, which is also present in ... ...
normal individuals with increasing age.

4.10

In Alzheimer's disease, the following neurochemical changes
occur:

    a Reduction in the amount of acetylcholine in the nucleus ... ...
basalis of Meynert.

    b Increase in the amount of dopamine metabolites in the ... ...
cortex.   ... ...

    c Reduction in noradrenaline in the cortex.   ... ...

    d Reduction in 5HT in the cortex.   ... ...

    e An increase in the amount of cortical neuropeptides such ... ...
as somatostatin.

Answers
4.7

a **True.** This damage of the septum pellucidum is particularly characteristic.
b **True.** Some of the clinical features resemble Parkinson's disease.
c **True.**
d **True.**
e **True.**

Lishman, W.A. (1998) *Organic psychiatry*, 3rd edn. Blackwell Science, Oxford, pp. 204–207.

4.8

a **True.**
b **True.**
c **True.**
d **True.**
e **True.**

Chick, J. and Cantwell, R. (eds.) (1994) *Seminars in alcohol and drug misuse*. Gaskell, London, p. 185.

4.9

a **False.** Frequently seen in Alzheimer's disease. They are eosinophilic rod-shaped structures which consist mainly of actin filaments.
b **True.** Found in Pick's disease, a rare cause of dementia.
c **False.** Mainly substantia nigra and locus coeruleus. Feature in 'Lewy body' dementia.
d **True.** These are occasionally found in normal elderly people. They are abundant in Alzheimer's disease.
e **True.** Mainly occur in the middle pyramidal layer of the hippocampus. Seen in Alzheimer's disease.

Puri, B. and Tyrer, P. (1992) *Sciences basic to psychiatry*. Churchill Livingstone, Edinburgh, pp. 175–176, 197.

4.10

a **True.** The enzymes for synthesis and degradation both being deficient.
b **False.** Reduction.
c **True.** Said to correlate with the severity of dementia at death.
d **True.** May be related to behavioural changes such as aggression and perhaps depression.
e **False.** Somatostatin is markedly reduced.

Lishman, W.A. (1998) *Organic psychiatry* , 3rd edn. Blackwell Science, Oxford , pp. 444–445.
Puri, B. and Tyrer, P. (1992) *Sciences basic to psychiatry*. Churchill Livingstone, Edinburgh, pp. 196–197.

Questions
4.11
[Certainty]

Phenylketonuria

	High	Med	Low
a Has an incidence of 1 per 1000 births in the UK.	...	...	...
b Is caused by a defective or absent DOPA decarboxylase enzyme.	...	...	...
c May be detected soon after birth by the Guthrie test.	...	...	...
d Requires that all phenylalanine be excluded from the diet.	...	...	...
e Sufferers should continue a restrictive diet into teenage years at least.	...	...	...

4.12
The following drugs are correctly paired with their class:

	High	Med	Low
a aliphatic phenothiazine—thioridazine.	...	...	...
b piperidine—sulpiride.	...	...	...
c piperazine—chlorpromazine.	...	...	...
d butylpiperidine—pimozide.	...	...	...
e dibenzodiazepine—clozapine.	...	...	...

4.13
Drugs which induce metabolizing enzymes in the liver include:

	High	Med	Low
a Chlorpromazine.	...	...	...
b Carbamazepine.	...	...	...
c Caffeine.	...	...	...
d Disulfiram.	...	...	...
e Sodium valproate.	...	...	...

4.14
The use of antipsychotic medication is associated with

	High	Med	Low
a A greater risk of parkinsonian side effects in older men compared to older women.	...	...	...
b Reduced side effects in patients with Lewy body dementia.	...	...	...
c Acute dystonia, best treated with oral procyclidine.	...	...	...
d Akathisia, best treated with beta blockers.	...	...	...
e Tardive dyskinesia, which is not related to the amount of neuroleptic exposure.	...	...	...

Answers
4.11

a **False.** 1 per 14 000 births.

b **False.** The enzyme at fault is phenylalanine hydroxylase.

c **True.** All newborn babies are screened in the UK.

d **False.** As phenylalanine is an essential amino acid, a very small amount is required to be included in the diet

e **True.**

Kendell, R.E. and Zealley, A.K. (eds.) (1993) *Companion to psychiatric studies*, 5th edn. Churchill Livingstone, Edinburgh, p. 632.

4.12

a **False.** aliphatic phenothiazine = chlorpromazine, promazine.

b **False.** piperidine = thioridazine.

c **False.** piperazine = trifluoperazine, fluphenazine.

d **True.**

e **True.**

Cookson, J., Crammer, J., and Heine, B. (1993) *The use of drugs in psychiatry*, 3rd edn. Gaskell, London, pp. 233–249.

4.13

a **True.** Chlorpromazine induces the enzymes that metabolises it resulting in some decrease in effectiveness of a given dose with time. It also inhibits liver metabolism of other some drugs.

b **True.**

c **True.**

d **False.** Disulfiram inhibits aldehyde dehydrogenase in the liver and hence the unpleasant effect with alcohol use.

e **False.** Sodium valproate inhibits liver enzymes metabolizing several compounds including phenytoin, carbamazepine, and phenobarbitone and so may cause toxicity.

Puri, B. and Tyrer, P. (1992) *Sciences basic to psychiatry*. Churchill Livingstone, Edinburgh, pp. 111–112

4.14

a **False.** Increased in women.

b **False.** Neuroleptic sensitivity can be markedly increased.

c **False.** Can be life-threatening, especially if respiratory muscles are affected. These situations require prompt treatment with intravenous procyclidine.

d **False.** Reduce the dose of neuroleptic first, if possible, then try beta-blockers or diazepam. Anticholinergics are usually of little benefit.

e **False.**

King, D. (ed.) (1995) *Seminars in clinical psychopharmacology*. Gaskell, London, pp. 282–287.

Questions

4.15

	[Certainty]		
The following statements regarding catecholamine synthesis and breakdown are true:	High	Med	Low
a The conversion of noradrenaline to adrenaline involves phenylethanolamine-*N*-methyl transferase.	...	...	...
b Catechol-*O*-methyltransferase is found in high concentrations in liver and kidney.	...	...	...
c Dopamine is catabolized to vanillylmandelic acid.	...	...	...
d Pseudocholinesterases are faster acting than true cholinesterases.	...	...	...
e Tyrosine hydroxylase is involved in the biosynthesis of serotonin.	...	...	...

4.16

The following statements regarding the electroencephalogram (EEG) are true:

	High	Med	Low
a Alpha EEG activity is attenuated by eye opening.	...	...	...
b EEG recording procedure is by convention, according to the 10–20 electrode system.	...	...	...
c Sleep spindles and K complexes occur during stage 3 of sleep.	...	...	...
d Dreaming is confined to rapid eye movement (REM) sleep.	...	...	...
e Intravenous thiopentone will reduce high frequency β activity.	...	...	...

4.17

Stimulation of the parasympathetic system causes

	High	Med	Low
a Slowing heart rate.	...	...	...
b Dilated pupils.	...	...	...
c Increased acid secretion in the stomach.	...	...	...
d Salivary secretion.	...	...	...
e Bronchodilation.	...	...	...

Answers
4.15

  a **True.**

  b **True.**

  c **False.** Dopamine is catabolized to homovanillic acid.

  d **False.** They are slower acting than true cholinesterases.

  e **False.** Tyrosine hydroxylase is involved in the biosynthesis of noradrenaline and adrenaline. Tryptophan hydroxylase is the rate limiting step in the biosynthesis of serotonin.

Note:

Tyrosine—(1)→DOPA—(2)→dopamine—(3)→noradrenaline—(4)→adrenaline

(1) Tyrosine hydroxylase

(2) DOPA decarboxylase

(3) Dopamine-β-hydroxylase

(4) Phenylethanolamine-N-methyl transferase

Puri, B. and Tyrer, P. (1992) *Sciences basic to psychiatry*. Churchill Livingstone, Edinburgh, pp. 95–103.

4.16

  a **True.** Alpha EEG activity is attenuated by eye opening and replaced by beta activity.

  b **True.** An international system using specific scalp landmarks.

  c **False.** Sleep spindles (12–14 Hz) and K complexes (large positive followed by large negative EEG deflection) occur during stage 2 of sleep.

  d **False.** Dreaming usually occurs in REM sleep but can occur in non-REM sleep.

  e **False.** Intravenous thiopentone will increase high frequency beta activity and reduce the risk of seizure.

Puri, B. and Tyrer, P. (1992) *Sciences basic to psychiatry*. Churchill Livingstone, Edinburgh, pp. 60–65.

4.17

  a **True.** The vagus (Xth) nerve descends from the dorsal nucleus to ganglions in the walls of the thoracic and abdominal viscera.

  b **False.** Pupillary constriction is controlled by the IIIrd cranial nerve, from the Edinger–Westphal nucleus via the ciliary ganglion to the sphincter pupillae. Atropine blocks the parasympathetic system.

  c **True.** Both the sympathetic and parasympathetic systems are regulated by the limbic system, hypothalamus, and reticular formation.

  d **True.** VIIth and IXth nerves.

  e **False.**

Lindsay, K., Bone, I., and Callander, R. (1991) *Neurology and neurosurgery illustrated*, 2nd edn. Churchill Livingstone, Edinburgh, pp. 439–441.

Questions
4.18   [Certainty]

Neuroendocrine abnormalities in psychiatry include: High   Med   Low

  a A failure by exogenous dexamethasone to suppress   ...   .
     cortisol only seen in melancholic depression.

  b Hypercortisolism and loss of cortisol diurnal rhythm in   ...   .
     anorexia nervosa.

  c Blunted cortisol and prolactin responses to serotonin   ...   .
     probes in obsessive–compulsive disorder.

  d The sick euthyroid picture in anorexia nervosa.   ...   .

  e Exaggerated growth hormone response in depression.   ...   .

4.19

The theory of mind

  a Is related to the anti-psychiatry movement.   ...   .

  b States that electroconvulsive therapy (ECT) is associated   ...   .
     with brain damage.

  c Develops at approximately 4 years of age.   ...   .

  d Is abnormal in autism.   ...   .

  e Refers to a child's hypotheses about a person's unseen   ...   .
     mental constructs.

4.20

The following are true:

  a The Minnesota Mutiphasic Personality Inventory   ...   .
     (MMPI) has 10 clinical subscales.

  b The thematic apperception test involves pairing pictures   ...   .
     and words.

  c The Wechsler Adult Intelligence Scale (WAIS) has   ...   .
     subtests including abstraction and visuospatial
     orientation.

  d Mental retardation corresponds with an IQ 1.5 SD below   ...   .
     the mean.

  e The Eysenck Personality Questionnaire (EPQ) includes a   ...   .
     lie scale.

Answers
4.18

   a **False.** There is a failure of suppression in the dexamethasone suppression test (DST) in depression, but early hopes that this would prove a trait marker have faded. For example, DST non-suppression is also seen in schizophrenia, anorexia, and alcoholism.

   b **False.** Hypercortisolism is found, but the cortisol diurnal rhythm is preserved.

   c **True.** This suggests a serotonin system subsensitivity. Abnormalities in the dopamine system have also been described in OCD.

   d **True.** The sick euthyroid syndrome consists of a low total T_4, normal free T_4, and low T_3.

   e **False.** There is a reduced growth hormone response (to levodopa) in depression. Blunted prolactin and TSH response to TRH are also observed.

Morgan, G and Butler, S. (eds.) (1993) *Seminars in basic neurosciences*. Gaskell, London, pp. 242–244.

4.19

   a **False.**
   b **False.**
   c **True.**
   d **True.**
   e **True.** A classic experiment to illustrate this is the 'deceptive box task'. A box of Smarties which contains pencils is presented to a child. Typically a child will predict that there are Smarties inside and will be surprised to see pencils. The majority of 4 year olds will correctly predict that the next child will think that there are Smarties in the box, whereas 3 year olds usually fail to do this.

Tantum, D. and Birchwood, M. (eds.) (1994) *Seminars in psychology and the social sciences*. Gaskell, London, pp. 16–20.

4.20

   a **True.**
   b **False.** Involves relating own story to ambiguous pictures.
   c **False.** Verbal and performance scales with 11 subtests.
   d **False.** 2 SDs for an IQ of 70 or less. One SD approximates to 15 IQ points. Mental retardation is suggested by an IQ of less than 70, i.e. 2 SD below the mean.
   e **True.** Measures three dimensions: E (extroversion), N (neuroticism), and P (psychotocism or 'tough mindedness').

Puri, B. and Tyrer, P. (1992) *Sciences basic to psychiatry*. Churchill Livingstone, Edinburgh, pp. 290–292.

Questions
4.21

In classical conditioning	High	Med	Low
a There must be a contingent relationship between the conditioned stimulus and the unconditioned stimulus.	...	...	...
b Voluntary behaviour is strengthened when paired with a reward.	...	...	...
c The time from the onset of the unconditioned stimulus to the onset of the conditioned response is called the latency.	...	...	...
d A generalization gradient may form with stimuli similar to the conditioned stimulus.	...	...	...
e Research is associated with the work of Pavlov and Skinner.	...	...	...

4.22

Regarding Piaget's stages of cognitive development:			
a External reality is not distinct from self in the sensorimotor stage.	...	...	...
b Objective conception is acquired early.	...	...	...
c Egocenticity characterizes the preoperational stage.	...	...	...
d The boundary between concrete and formal operational stages is not clear.	...	...	...
e Hypothesizing is not achieved till 7 years old.	...	...	...

4.23

In group processes			
a Conformity and communication have been routinely found to be associated with increased cohesiveness.	...	...	...
b Cohesiveness refers to how attractive a group is to its members.	...	...	...
c Groups composed of individuals who are also members of many other groups are likely to show increased cohesiveness.	...	...	...
d Spontaneously formed groups often turn out to be low in cohesiveness.	...	...	...
e Conformity to norms is a cause of group cohesiveness.	...	...	...

Answers
4.21

a **True.**

b **False.** This is Thorndike's 'law of effect' and is associated with operant conditioning.

c **False.** Latency is the time from onset of the conditioned stimulus to the onset of the conditioned response.

d **True.**

e **False.** Skinner is associated with operant conditioning research.

Note: Learning theory is made more difficult by a large amount of jargon, However, this is important to know.

Puri, B. and Tyrer, P. (1992) *Sciences basic to psychiatry*. Churchill Livingstone, Edinburgh, pp. 279–280.

4.22

a **True.** In the sensorimotor stage (age 0–2 years) there is difficulty conceiving of objects not present, and perception is subordinate to action. That is, external reality (and self) are defined in terms of the infant's own actions.

b **False.** Before the age of 7, Piaget felt that the child is egocentric, unable to logically reason, and under the sway of the superficial perceived image.

c **True.** During the preoperational stage (aged 2–7 years) the child is thought to be egocentric; capable of non-logical thought and distinguishing between self and not-self; but fails to recognize conservation of different quantities.

d **True.** One of the criticisms levelled at Piaget is that many adults do not reason solely in the formal operational way. The young child appears to be more competent than Piaget had supposed, whereas the adult is less so.

e **False.** Hypothesising is a characteristic of the formal operational stage, which Piaget felt began at 12 years old.

Tantum, D. and Birchwood, M. (eds.) (1994) *Seminars in psychology and the social sciences*. Gaskell, London, pp. 3–16.

4.23

a **True.**

b **True.**

c **False.** Due to competing interests.

d **True.**

e **True.**

Henry, C.L. (1973) *An introduction to social Psychology*, 2nd edn. Wiley, New York, pp. 329–347.

Questions
4.24
[Certainty]

The following factors are important in good leadership:

	High	Med	Low
a Contributing to the group goal.	...	...	...
b Laissez-faire supervision.	...	...	...
c Structuring a specific job.	...	...	...
d A considerate style in a boring job.	...	...	...
e An autocratic rather than participative approach.	...	...	...

4.25

Social expectations of illness include:

	High	Med	Low
a Exemption from normal role responsibilities, which must be legitimized.	...	...	...
b That care of those who are ill must be undertaken.	...	...	...
c The ill person should be under an obligation to get well.	...	...	...
d The doctor treating the ill person should be technically competent.	...	...	...
e An expectation that society will pay for the care of those ill.	...	...	...

Clinical

4.26

In the drug treatment of Parkinson's disease

	High	Med	Low
a Levodopa improves tremor more than rigidity and bradykinesia.	...	...	...
b Early treatment with selegiline will delay the need for levodopa therapy.	...	...	...
c Carbidopa is a peripheral dopa decarboxlase inhibitor.	...	...	...
d Bromocriptine acts by directly stimulating acetylcholine receptors.	...	...	...
e Amantadine is useful in drug-induced extrapyramidal syndromes.	...	...	...

Answers
4.24

a **True.** Leader status increases proportional to the contribution towards the group goal.

b **False.** Both laissez-faire and autocratic styles are less effective than a participative approach.

c **False.** Structuring involves setting standards and giving tasks, and is good when the job is unclear, but bad when the job is specific.

d **True.** The leadership behavioural factor of consideration is exemplified by a concern for others' opinion, and leads to a more satisfied group. This is particularly helpful in a boring or unclear job.

e **False.** See above. Also a democratic rather than authoritarian approach is thought to be beneficial.

Corsini, R.J. (ed.) (1984) *Encyclopaedia of psychology*, Vol. 2, pp. 282–286. Wiley, New York, Chichester.

4.25

a **True.** Parsons formulated illness as a social role—'the sick role'—which exempted the individual from normal social role responsibilities. This exemption was not automatic, and had to be legitimized. In industrialized societies the doctor is the key arbiter of this.

b **True.** While the illness lasts the sufferer is not expected to help themselves.

c **True.** The state of being ill is defined as being undesirable, and the ill person should want to get well.

d **False.** Although society may well expect this of its doctors, it is not an expectation of illness. However,, the ill person is obliged to seek technically competent help, and cooperate in the treatment process.

e **False.** Different societies have differing value systems.

Tantum, D. and Birchwood, M. (eds.) (1994) *Seminars in psychology and the social sciences*. Gaskell, London, pp. 319–320.

Clinical

4.26

a **False.** Levodopa improves rigidity and bradykinesia more than tremor.

b **False.** There is no convincing evidence for this.

c **True.**

d **False.** Bromocriptine acts by directly stimulating surviving dopamine receptors.

e **False.** Amantadine improves bradykinesia, tremor, and rigidity. It is relatively free from side effects.

British National Formulary, Section 4.9.1.

Questions
4.27

	[Certainty]		
Huntington's disease	High	Med	Low
a Is associated with abnormality of chromosome 5.	...	...	...
b Has a prevalence of 5 per 10 000 population in the UK.	...	...	...
c Is associated with memory deficits which are apparent early in the course of the illness.	...	...	...
d Is associated with caudate atrophy seen at neuroimaging.	...	...	...
e Is characteristically associated with a short illness course.	...	...	...

4.28

Narcolepsy
a Is characterized by an irresistible desire to sleep during the day.	...	...	...
b Is associated with catalepsy.	...	...	...
c Is familial in about one third of cases.	...	...	...
d Is associated with the human leukocyte antigen (HLA) B8.	...	...	...
e Is usually associated with absent REM sleep.	...	...	...

4.29

Korsakoff's syndrome
a Is invariably associated with alcohol abuse.	...	...	...
b Is reversible with high dose thiamine treatment.	...	...	...
c Causes extensive anterograde amnesia.	...	...	...
d Is associated with near normal primary memory.	...	...	...
e Is associated with characteristic pathological lesions in the periventricular and periaquaductal grey matter.	...	...	...

Answers
4.27

a **False.** The gene mutation lies on the short arm of chromosome 4.
b **False.** Approximately 5 per 100 000.
c **True.** Can be demonstrated clearly even within a year of onset of the chorea.
d **True.**
e **False.** It is associated with a longer course of illness than are other primary dementias.

Lishman, W.A. (1998) *Organic psychiatry*, 3rd edn. Blackwell Science, Oxford, pp. 465–471.

4.28

a **True.**
b **False.** Narcolepsy is associated with cataplexy. Cataplexy is a sudden collapse or loss of tone associated with strong emotion. The onset is usually under 30 years, and males are more frequently affected. Catalepsy is a stereotyped movement disorder seen in catatonia.
c **True.**
d **False.** Narcolepsy has been specifically associated with the DR2 and DQ subtype of the human leukocyte antigen.
e **False.** There is rapid onset of REM during daytime and nocturnal sleep.

Note: Gelineau's syndrome is the tetrad of narcolepsy, cataplexy, sleep paralysis, and hypnagogic hallucinations. Other sleep disorders of interest are the Kleine–Levin syndrome, and hypersomnia due to obstructive sleep apnoea. Night terrors and somnambulism are typically seen in children.

Lishman, W.A. (1998) *Organic psychiatry*, 3rd edn. Blackwell Science, Oxford, pp. 721–725.
Parkes, J.D. (1985) *Sleep and its disorders*. Saunders, London, pp. 617–632.

4.29

a **False.**
b **False.**
c **False.** There is extensive retrograde amnesia and a temporal gradient is often present.
d **True.** Korsakoff's syndrome is defined as an impairment of memory and learning out of proportion to other cognitive dysfunction. It may follow on from Wernicke's encephalopathy, or have a more insidious onset. Wernike's encephalopathy is thought to be caused by thiamine deficiency but treatment rarely reverses the memory deficit of Korsakoff's syndrome.
e **True.**

Note: Wernicke's encephalopathy consists of opthalmoplegia, confusion, and ataxia, due to thiamine deficiency secondary not only to alcoholism but other causes such as hyperemesis.

Kopelman, M. D. (1995) The Korsakoff syndrome. *British Journal of Psychiatry* 166, 154–173.

Questions
4.30
[Certainty]

Compared to classical Creutzfeldt–Jakob disease (CJD), characteristics of new variant CJD are

	High	Med	Low
a Older age of onset.	...	...	...
b Shorter period between diagnosis and death.	...	...	...
c More psychiatric presenting features.	...	...	...
d More prion protein amyloid plaques.	...	...	...
e Only occurs in those eating beef.	...	...	...

4.31
Regarding affective disorder:

a The occurrence of severe depressive illness in Japan has been shown to be considerably lower than that in the UK.	...	...	...
b An increased frequency of obsessional traits has been found in the personalities of those with depressive illnesses.	...	...	...
c The lifetime prevalence of bipolar affective disorder has been found to be 1–2%.	...	...	...
d Tetrabenazine acts as an effective antidepressant.	...	...	...
e L-DOPA has been shown to enhance the antidepressant effect of MAOIs.	...	...	...

4.32
With regard to life events and vulnerability factors in depression

a The presence of 'search after meaning' makes it more difficult to assess the importance of recent life events in the aetiology of depression.	...	...	...
b According to Brown and Harris, the loss of one's mother before the age of 11 is shown to directly affect the likelihood of developing a depressive illness.	...	...	...
c The Islington survey identified low self esteem as the most important vulnerability factor.	...	...	...
d High expressed emotion in the family has been shown to lead to a much greater risk of relapse in depression.	...	...	...
e After hysterectomy the risk of depression in those with normal pelvic pathology is much higher than in those with abnormalities.	...	...	...

Answers
4.30

a **False.** Younger age of onset, i.e. 19–39 years for new variant compared with 50–70 years for classical CJD.

b **False.** More insidious onset and longer course.

c **True.** Such as anxiety and depression.

d **True.**

e **False.** The link with eating beef remains controversial; others working with animal products may also be at risk.

Harrison, P.J. (1997) BSE and human prion disease. *British Journal of Psychiatry* 170, 298–300.

4.31

a **False.** A WHO study which included Basle, Montreal, Teheran, Nagasaki, and Tokyo found no significant differences.

b **True.** They have been found to be introverted, obsessional, and dependant.

c **True.** It is approximately 4.4% for major depression.

d **False.** Tetrabenazine and reserpine deplete MAO storage vesicles and may cause severe depression.

e **True.** It may even precipitate hypomania.

Kendell, R.E. and Zealley, A.K. (eds.) (1993) *Companion to psychiatric studies*, 5th edn. Churchill Livingstone, Edinburgh, pp. 427–459.

4.32

a **True.**

b **False.** This is a 'vulnerability factor' and also requires a ' provoking agent'.

c **True.** A survey of 400 working class women aged 18–50 with at least one child under 18 at home.

d **True.** Similar to schizophrenia.

e **True.** There is a link with previous psychiatric disorder and absence of pelvic pathology.

Gelder, M., Gath, D., Mayou, R., and Cowen, P. (eds.) (1996) *The Oxford textbook of psychiatry*, 3rd edn. Oxford University Press, Oxford, pp. 215–219.

Kendell, R.E. and Zealley, A.K. (eds.) (1993) *Companion to psychiatric studies*, 5th edn. Churchill Livingstone, Edinburgh, pp. 427–459.

Questions
4.33

The following statements are correct:	High	Med	Low
a de Clerambault's syndrome is characterized by delusional jealousy.	...	...	...
b Schizoaffective disorder is a term coined by Kahlbaum.	...	...	...
c Once admitted to psychiatric hospital migrants are at greater risk of being labelled as schizophrenic.	...	...	...
d Parents of schizophrenics are more often psychiatrically disturbed than parents of unaffected children.	...	...	...
e Siblings of schizophrenics show an excess of winter births (in the northern hemisphere).	...	...	...

4.34

In those suffering from schizophrenia			
a Family dynamics are not significant in the likelihood of relapse of symptoms.	...	...	...
b Positive symptoms are more amenable to drug treatment than negative symptoms.	...	...	...
c The Brief Psychiatric Rating Scale (BPRS) is a useful measure of overall psychopathology.	...	...	...
d The P300 event-related potential in response to an external sensory stimulus is abnormally reduced in latency.	...	...	...
e Abnormal eye-tracking is described.	...	...	...

4.35

Associations of anxiety disorder include:			
a Mitral valve lesions found in over 75% of sufferers.	...	...	...
b The most common change of diagnosis to depression.	...	...	...
c High thoracic breathing in the hyperventilation syndrome.	...	...	...
d A bimodal peak of onset in agoraphobia.	...	...	...
e Social phobia being commoner among females.	...	...	...

Answers
4.33

a **False.** de Clerambault's syndrome is also known as erotomania. The subject (usually female) is deluded that another (usually a man of higher social standing) is in love with her.

b **False.** Kasanin.

c **True.**

d **True.**

e **False.**

Kendell, R.E. and Zealley, A.K. (eds.) (1993) *Companion to psychiatric studies*, 5th edn. Churchill Livingstone, Edinburgh, pp. 397–423, 459–462, 468–469.

4.34

a **False.** The amount of expressed emotion (EE) by a patient's family is particularly important in the relapse of schizophrenia.

b **True.** Although claims have been made for 'newer' antipsychotics such as clozapine and risperidone for having beneficial effects on negative symptoms.

c **True.** The BPRS is a global symptom rating scale with subcomponents measuring both subjective and observer variables.

d **False.** P300 changes include reduced amplitude and prolonged latency. These findings have been claimed to be a marker of genetic vulnerability to schizophrenia.

e **True.** Abnormality in smooth pursuit eye movements are described.

Kendell, R.E. and Zealley, A.K. (eds.) (1993) *Companion to psychiatric studies*, 5th edn. Churchill Livingstone, Edinburgh, pp. 397–423.

4.35

a **False.** Up to one third of sufferers.

b **False.** Alcoholism is the commonest diagnosis.

c **True.**

d **True.** Which occurs in the late teens and mid thirties.

e **False.** Equal sex incidence.

Gelder, M., Gath, D., Mayou, R., and Cowen, P. (eds.) (1996) *The Oxford textbook of psychiatry*, 3rd edn. Oxford University Press, Oxford, pp. 163–169.

Kendell, R.E. and Zealley, A.K. (eds.) (1993) *Companion to psychiatric studies*, 5th edn. Churchill Livingstone, Edinburgh, pp. 498–502.

Questions

4.36
[Certainty]

The following statements regarding psychogenic amnesia are true:
                                                High Med Low

   a It is usually of gradual onset.   ...   .
   b It should only be diagnosed in the absence of organic   ...   .
      disease.
   c Total personal amnesia with preservation of reading and   ...   .
      writing skills is in keeping with the diagnosis.
   d Recovery is often incomplete.   ...   .
   e Vague wandering is a recognized feature.   ...   .

4.37

In the pharmacological treatment of schizophrenia
   a After the first episode it is suggested that cautious   ...   .
      withdrawal of medication is attempted if the patient has
      remained well for 1 year.
   b Clozapine offers proven advantage over other drugs in   ...   .
      treatment-resistant schizophrenia.
   c Among those who adhere fully to treatment, 40% will   ...   .
      relapse each year.
   d Haloperidol can be administered intravenously to acutely   ...   .
      agitated patients.
   e Substituted benzamides are preferred for poorly   ...   .
      compliant patients.

4.38

Tardive dyskinesia
   a Affects approximately one third of patients who are   ...   .
      chronically ingesting antipsychotics.
   b Is prevented by 'drug holidays'.   ...   .
   c Includes the 'Pisa syndrome'.   ...   .
   d Is more likely in those patients who suffer from affective   ...   .
      disorders.
   e Can be treated with tetrabenazine.   ...   .

4.39

The following are used as anti-epileptics:
   a Clonazepam.   ...   .
   b Acetazolamide.   ...   .
   c Piracetam.   ...   .
   d Gabapentin.   ...   .
   e Topiramate.   ...   .

Answers
4.36

a **False.** Usually a sudden onset of memory impairment.

b **True.**

c **True.** The most common type is failure to recall events during a circumscribed period of time.

d **False.** Onset and end are usually sudden. Recovery is usually complete and recurrences uncommon.

e **True.** Wandering is usually vague in psychogenic amnesia. In fugue states wandering tends to be more purposeful.

Kendell, R.E. and Zealley, A.K. (eds.) (1993) *Companion to psychiatric studies*, 5th edn. Churchill Livingstone, Edinburgh, p. 514.

4.37

a **True.**

b **True.**

c **False.** 10%.

d **True.** Although it is not a 'tranquillizer' of first choice. Note intravenous procyclidine should be given (in a separate syringe) at the same time to counter the almost inevitable extrapyramidal effects.

e **False.** These (e.g. sulpiride) have to be given orally and therefore rely on a greater degree of compliance from the patient, although their side-effect profile is probably better than many alternatives.

Cookson, J., Crammer, J., and Heine, B. (1993) *The use of drugs in psychiatry*, 3rd edn. Gaskell, London, pp. 97–111.

4.38

a **False.** Approximately 20%.

b **False.** 'Drug holidays', i.e. drug-free periods interrupting chronic treatment, do not prevent, and may even enhance, the development of tardive dyskinesia.

c **True.** Otherwise known as asymmetrical axial dystonia.

d **True.** Also more likely in the elderly, those with organic brain damage, and those who exhibit other extrapyramidal side effects early on in treatment.

e **True.** Tetrabenazine depletes presynaptic dopamine storage granules and is worth trying in patients with severe symptoms.

Kendell, R.E. and Zealley, A.K. (eds.) (1993) *Companion to psychiatric studies*, 5th edn. Churchill Livingstone, Edinburgh, p. 823.

4.39

a **True.** Used for all forms of epilepsy, myoclonus, and status epilepticus.

b **True.** A carbonic anhydrase inhibitor used as second line treatment for tonic clonic and partial seizures.

c **True.** Used as an adjunctive treatment for myoclonus.

d **True.** Used as an adjunctive treatment for partial epilepsy.

e **True.** Used as an adjunctive treatment for partial epilepsy.

British National Formulary, Section 4.5

Questions

4.40

	[Certainty]		
Phenytoin	High	Med	Low
a Is eliminated by zero-order kinetics.	...	...	...
b Causes hypercalcaemia.	...	...	...
c Has a high therapeutic index.	...	...	...
d Side-effects include a microcytic anaemia.	...	...	...
e Can be administered intravenously.	...	...	...

4.41

Maternal serum markers suggestive of a diagnosis of Down's syndrome at 16 weeks' gestation include:

a Raised human chorionic gonadotropin.	...	...	...
b Raised α-fetoprotein.	...	...	...
c Lowered C-reactive protein.	...	...	...
d Lowered unconjugated oestriol.	...	...	...
e Raised chorioembryonic antigen.	...	...	...

4.42

Regarding hyperkinetic disorder of childhood

a The onset must be before the age of 6 in order to make a diagnosis, according to ICD 10.	...	...	...
b Pervasive hyperactivity is sufficient to make the diagnosis.	...	...	...
c The prevalence is 1–2% in the UK.	...	...	...
d The side effects of treatment with methylphenidate include insomnia and weight gain.	...	...	...
e Approximately 30% of sufferers may show residual symptoms in adulthood.	...	...	...

4.43

The following are major features of infantile autism:

a Onset before 30 months.	...	...	...
b Alexithymia.	...	...	...
c Reliance on gesture rather than language.	...	...	...
d Minor physical anomalies.	...	...	...
e Approximately equal rates in boys and girls.	...	...	...

Answers
4.40

  a **True.** This means that it has saturable metabolism. This has implications for the way it should be increased as therapeutic levels are approached, i.e. not more than 25 mg at a time.

  b **False.** Causes hypocalcaemia and rickets.

  c **False.** Has a low therapeutic index which means that there is a narrow margin between therapeutic and toxic levels.

  d **False.** Side effects include megaloblastic anaemia due to folate malabsorption

  e **True.** To gain rapid control of status epilepticus after diazepam administration. Electrocardiogam (ECG) and blood pressure monitoring should be performed as intravenous phenytoin can cause arrhythmias.

British National Formulary, Section 4.8

4.41

  a **True.**

  b **False.** This is suggestive of a neural tube defect or a multiple pregnancy. A low α-fetoprotein level is suggestive of Down's syndrome.

  c **False.**

  d **True.**

  e **False.**

Note: The finding of raised human chorionic gonadotropin, lowered α-fetoprotein, and lowered unconjugated oestriol is the so-called 'triple test' used at 16 weeks.

Mueller, R.F. and Young, I.D. (1995) *Emery's elements of medical genetics*, 9th edn. Churchill Livingstone, Edinburgh, pp. 269–271.

4.42

  a **True.**

  b **False.** Also decreased attention and distractibility.

  c **False.** Under 0.1% prevalence. Quoted as up to 1–2% in the US.

  d **False.** Decreased growth and appetite are side effects.

  e **True.** These include aggressive behaviour and educational underachievement.

Hoare, P. (1993) *Essential child psychiatry*. Churchill Livingstone, Edinburgh, pp. 164–174.

4.43

  a **True.** Developmental abnormalities must be present in the first 3 years of life to allow the diagnosis.

  b **False.** A lack of emotional response to other people's verbal and non-verbal overtures is often seen, but this cannot be described as alexithymia.

  c **False.** As well as abnormal language development, including a tendency to echolalia and pronoun reversal, there is a lack of gesture and mime.

  d **False.** Although there may be associated disorders, such as fragile X and tuberous sclerosis, there is no characteristic body habitus or phenotype.

  e **False.** 3–4 times more common in boys than girls.

World Health Organization (1992) *Tenth revision of the International Classification of Disease (ICD 10)*. WHO, Geneva, pp. 252–255.

Questions
4.44

Regarding parole:

		High	Med	Low
a	It is the system of early release from prison.	...	...	...
b	It may be granted after serving 50% of a sentence of 4 years or more.	...	...	...
c	It is not associated with statutory provision for supervision after release.	...	...	...
d	The discretionary lifer parole panel always contains a psychiatrist.	...	...	...
e	It was introduced at the beginning of the twentieth century.	...	...	...

4.45

The following statements are true:

a	The term 'diminished responsibility' may be used in a charge of manslaughter.	...	...	...
b	'Actus rea' means guilty mind.	...	...	...
c	Epilepsy is an example of a sane automatism.	...	...	...
d	'Mens rea' may be affected by drug ingestion.	...	...	...
e	A hospital order can be made on the recommendation of one medical practitioner.	...	...	...

4.46

Physical complications of bereavement include:

a	Decreased growth hormone secretion.	...	...	...
b	Lowered serum prolactin.	...	...	...
c	Impairment of the immune response system.	...	...	...
d	Increased mortality from cardiovascular disease.	...	...	...
e	Increased adrenocortical activity.	...	...	...

4.47

The following statements are true:

a	Wernicke's encephalopathy is a treatable condition.	...	...	...
b	Chlorpromazine is an acceptable treatment in the acute phase of alcohol withdrawal.	...	...	...
c	Alcoholic hallucinosis is characterized by auditory hallucinations in the majority of cases.	...	...	...
d	Alcohol dependence is recognized under the Mental Health Act as reasonable grounds for short-term detention in hospital.	...	...	...
e	Men are more vulnerable to alcohol-related liver disease than women.	...	...	...

Answers
4.44
a **True.**
b **True.**
c **False.** Supervision is undertaken by a probation officer.
d **True.** As well as a judge and a layman who may be a criminologist or psychologist, etc.
e **False.** 1967.

Chiswick, D. and Cope R. (eds.) (1995) *Seminars in forensic psychiatry.* Gaskell, London, pp. 264–265.

4.45
a **False.** This term may only be used in a charge of murder.
b **False.** This is the actual act.
c **False.** Sane automatisms include confusional states and hypoglycaemia.
d **True.** Drugs may affect decision-making.
e **False.** Two doctors are required.

Chiswick, D. and Cope R. (eds.) (1995) *Seminars in forensic psychiatry.* Gaskell, London, pp. 114, 121, 124.

4.46
a **False.** Growth hormone secretion is increased.
b **False.** Serum prolactin is raised.
c **True.**
d **True.** Especially in widowers.
e **True.**

Note: Similar to other situations that cause distress and depression, bereavement, and loss cause a variety of physiological responses.

Parkes, C.M. (1998) Coping with loss: bereavement in adult life. *British Medical Journal* 316, 856–859.

4.47
a **True.** Often cited as a psychiatric emergency. Prompt treatment with intravenous thiamine is essential to prevent further neurological damage and progression to Korsakoff's syndrome.
b **False.** It will reduce the seizure threshold and make seizures more likely.
c **True.** Delirium tremens is associated with visual hallucinations. Alcoholic hallucinosis is characterized by auditory hallucinations.
d **False.** Alcohol and substance dependence, along with personality disorder, are not *per se* grounds for detention under the Mental Health Act. However, these conditions can be associated with other mental illnesses which themselves are grounds for detention.
e **False.** The converse is true.

British National Formulary, Section 9.6.2,

Kendell, R.E. and Zealley, A.K. (eds.) (1993) *Companion to psychiatric studies*, 5th edn. Churchill Livingstone, Edinburgh, pp. 377–380.

Questions

4.48

[Certainty]

'Harm reduction' in terms of illicit drug use includes the following concepts:

	High	Med	Low
a Reduction or stopping of drug use.	...	...	...
b If using, reduce or stop injecting.	...	...	...
c If sharing needles, clean the injecting equipment first.	...	...	...
d Education on safer sex.	...	...	...
e Immunization against hepatitis B.	...	...	...

4.49

Cognitive analytical therapy (CAT):

	High	Med	Low
a Begins by agreeing goals of therapy and setting time limits.	...	...	...
b Is intended to apply cognitive techniques within a framework of psychoanalytic understanding.	...	...	...
c Differs from cognitive therapy in focusing more on specific patterns of thinking and less on interpersonal behaviour.	...	...	...
d Differs from psychoanalytical therapy in focusing less on the transference.	...	...	...
e Differs from psychoanalytical therapy in focusing more on identifying defence mechanisms.	...	...	...

4.50

The following statements are correct:

	High	Med	Low
a The repertory grid is a useful test of frontal lobe function.	...	...	...
b Kelly's personal construct therapy allows the subject to evaluate significant relationships in their past and present lives.	...	...	...
c Sensitivity groups evolved from the work of Lewin's T-groups.	...	...	...
d Rogerian therapy is a directive form of therapy.	...	...	...
e Carl Jung is associated with ideas regarding encounter therapy.	...	...	...

Answers
4.48

  a **True.**
  b **True.**
  c **True.**
  d **True.**
  e **True.**

Note: Other aims include, if injecting, to reduce or stop sharing and to avoid contaminated equipment. Other strategies include education on risks of injection and overdose, how to clean injecting equipment, provision of needles and condoms, HIV testing, and substitute oral drugs.

Chick, J. and Cantwell, R. (eds.) (1994) *Seminars in alcohol and drug misuse*. Gaskell, London, pp. 39–40.

4.49

  a **True.** As is the case with most psychological therapies.
  b **True.**
  c **False.** CAT differs from cognitive therapy in focusing less on specific patterns of thinking and more on interpersonal behaviour and the formulation of assumptions that lie behind them.
  d **True.**
  e **False.** CAT focuses less on identifying defence mechanisms and less on the transference.

Gelder, M., Gath, D., Mayou, R., and Cowen, P. (eds.) (1996) *The Oxford textbook of psychiatry*, 3rd edn. Oxford University Press, Oxford, pp. 612–613.

4.50

  a **False.** The repertory grid studies the cognitive constructs underlying significant relationships in the subjects past and present life.
  b **True.**
  c **True.**
  d **False.** Rogerian therapy is a non-directive form of therapy. It is also known as client-centred therapy.
  e **False.** Carl Jung is associated with the collective unconscious, archetypes, and the anima/animus.

Brown, D. and Pedder, J. (1991) *Introduction to psychotherapy*, 2nd edn. Routledge, London, pp. 166–167, 178.

Paper 5: Questions

Basic science

5.1

Magnetic resonance imaging (MRI) of the brain:

	High	Med	Low
a Involves using ionizing radiation to study structure.	...	...	...
b Shows bony structures clearer than computed tomography (CT) scans.	...	...	...
c Is less expensive than CT scanning.	...	...	...
d Takes a shorter period of time than CT scanning.	...	...	...
e Is of little use in examination of brain stem lesions because of excessive artefact from surrounding bone.	...	...	...

5.2

The following neuroanatomical statements are true:

a The Sylvian fissure (lateral sulcus) separates the frontal and parietal lobes.	...	...	...
b The central sulcus separates frontal and temporal lobes.	...	...	...
c The hypothalamus is a mesencephalic structure.	...	...	...
d The cerebral cortex is comprised of six layers of nerve cells.	...	...	...
	...	...	...
e The caudate nucleus is comprised of the globus pallidus and the lentiform.	...	...	...

5.3

Left-handed people are

a Mostly right hemisphere dominant for speech.	...	...	...
b More commonly twins than the general population.	...	...	...
c More likely than expected to develop schizophrenia.	...	...	...
d Known to have a more asymmetric brain than right handers.	...	...	...
e More prone to affective disorder than right handers.	...	...	...

Paper 5: Answers

Basic science

5.1

a **False.** No ionizing radiation is used, unlike computed tomography (CT) scanning.

b **False.** Bone contains little water and therefore returns only a small signal on MRI, in contrast to CT scanning which shows bone clearly.

c **False.** It is more costly.

d **False.** May take up to 1 hour depending on tissue being examined.

e **False.** There is little bony artefact and therefore is particularly useful for examining the brainstem and posterior fossa of the cranial cavity.

Kendell, R.E. and Zealley, A.K. (eds.) (1993) *Companion to psychiatric studies*, 5th edn. Churchill Livingstone, Edinburgh, pp. 476–480.

5.2

a **False.** The Sylvian fissure separates the frontal and temporal lobes.

b **False.** The central sulcus separates frontal and parietal lobes

c **False.** Diencephalic structures include thalamus, hypothalamus, subthalamus, epithalamus, and pituitary. Mesencephalic structures cerebellum, pons, and medulla. Metencephalic structures include tectum, corpora quadragemini, cerebral aqueduct, and basis pedunculis. Telencephalic structures include the cerebral hemispheres and corpus striatum.

d **True.** From surface downward the layers are; molecular, outer granular, outer pyramidal, inner granular, inner pyramidal, and fusiform.

e **False.** The lentiform nucleus is the shape of a biconvex lens and is made up of the globus pallidus (medially) and the putamen (laterally).

Kendell, R.E. and Zealley, A.K. (eds.) (1993) *Companion to psychiatric studies*, 5th edn. Churchill Livingstone, Edinburgh, pp. 99–100.

McMinn, R.M.H. (1994) *Last's anatomy, regional and applied*, 9th edn. Churchill Livingstone, Edinburgh, pp. 577–578, 581–582.

5.3

a **False.** About 70% have speech lateralized to the left (dominant) hemisphere.

b **True.** Roughly 20% compared to 9%. Theories for this include fetal crowding and mirroring.

c **False.** Early reports suggested this was the case, but now the consensus is that mixed handedness, rather than fully left lateralized, is more common. This may be due to minimal brain damage, or possibly to Crow's theory of a failure in the lateralization process being linked to the gene(s) for schizophrenia.

d **False.** Usually less anatomically and functionally asymmetric.

e **False.** Although the right hemisphere is meant to be important in emotional and non-verbal processing, there is no evidence to support this.

Springer, S. and Deutsch, G. (1981) *Left brain, right brain*. Freeman, San Francisco, pp. 103–121.

Questions

5.4

	[Certainty]		
Concerning speech disorder:	High	Med	Low
a Damage to the superior temporal gyrus causes Wernicke's aphasia.	...	...	...
b Prosody is dependent on intact left hemisphere function.	...	...	...
c Lesions in the cerebellar vermis and paravermis lead to an ataxic dysarthria.	...	...	...
d Logoclonia occurs in extrapyramidal disease.	...	...	...
e Aphonia usually has a psychogenic basis.	...	...	...

5.5

The following are associated with temporal lobe lesions:			
a Astereognosis.	...	...	...
b Cortical deafness.	...	...	...
c Homonymous lower quadrantanopia.	...	...	...
d Amnesic syndromes.	...	...	...
e Alexia.	...	...	...

5.6

Wernicke's encephalopathy may result from:			
a Carbon monoxide poisoning.	...	...	...
b Heavy metal poisoning.	...	...	...
c Cerebral tumours.	...	...	...
d Anaesthetic accidents.	...	...	...
e Bilateral hippocampal damage.	...	...	...

Answers

5.4

a **True.** Wernicke's area is Brodmann area 22, which is at the posterior end of the Sylvian fissure (i.e. the temporoparietal region) on the lateral surface of the left hemisphere, in right-handers and many left-handers. The receptive dysphasia implies that the spoken word is understood and the appropriate reply or action initiated.

b **False.** Prosody is the emotional inflection in speech, and is a non-dominant hemisphere function. Thus the non-dominant hemisphere cannot simply be viewed as the non-verbal hemisphere.

c **True.** Otherwise known as 'scanning speech' (monotonous and staccato in quality) and often seen in multiple sclerosis and Friedreich's ataxia.

d **True.** Logoclonia involves the spastic repetition of syllables, and the patient may get stuck on a particular word. Similar to palilalia, where there is repetition of the last word or words in a patient's speech.

e **False.** A complete inability to produce sound or only being able to vocalize in a whisper (a 'stage whisper') may be due to paralysis of both vocal cords (e.g. by medullary infarct) or motor neurone disease. Occasionally it may be dissociative in origin (F44.4 in ICD 10).

Morgan, G and Butler, S. (eds.) (1993) *Seminars in basic neurosciences*. Gaskell, London, pp. 26–33.

5.5

a **False.** Parietal sensory cortex.

b **True.** Temporal auditory cortex. Cortical blindness is localized to the occipital lesions.

c **False.** Lower quadrantanopia is parietal optic radiation, upper quadrantanopia is temporal.

d **True.** Bilateral medial temporal lobe. Remember the Kluver–Bucy syndrome.

e **True.** Alexia and agraphia are seen in posterior dominant temporal lobe lesions.

Crimlisk, H. and Taylor, M. (1996) MRCPsych: How to cope with a neuropsychiatric case. *British Journal of Hospital Medicine* 56, 103–107.

5.6

a **True.**

b **True.**

c **True.**

d **True.**

e **True.**

Puri, B. and Tyrer, P. (1992) *Sciences basic to psychiatry*. Churchill Livingstone, Edinburgh, p. 195.

Questions

5.7

Imprinting

	High	Med	Low
a Is irreversible.	...	...	...
b Is limited to a very brief period.	...	...	...
c Is generally limited to birds.	...	...	...
d When 'abnormal' is a reason why animals reared in captivity have difficulty mating.	...	...	...
e Does not occur in humans.	...	...	...

5.8

The following statements are true:

a Intelligence quotient (IQ) distribution follows a Gaussian distribution.	...	...	...
b Subcultural retardation is greatest in social classes IV and V.	...	...	...
c Emotional deprivation may give rise to apparent retardation.	...	...	...
d Around 15% of those with learning disabilities have severe or profound handicap.	...	...	...
e Down's syndrome occurs at a rate of 3 per 1000 live births.	...	...	...

5.9

According to Chomsky

a Linguistic grammar is innate, and species-specific.	...	...	...
b All languages have a deep syntax in common.	...	...	...
c Cognitive development precedes language acquisition.	...	...	...
d Parapraxes are a form of fluent aphasia.	...	...	...
e Language determines thought.	...	...	...

Answers

5.7

a **True.**

b **True.** So-called 'critical' or 'sensitive' period.

c **False.** Seen throughout the animal kingdom.

d **True.** E.g. pandas having difficulty mating may be due to abnormal imprinting with humans during the period after their own birth.

e **False.**

Weller, M. and Eysenck, M. (1991) *The scientific basis of psychiatry*, 2nd edn. Saunders, Philadelphia, pp. 444–445.

5.8

a **False.** There are more people at the lower end of the distribution with an IQ of less than 70.

b **True.**

c **True.** Children need emotional and sensory stimulation to achieve maximum potential.

d **False.** Under 6% of those with learning disabilities are severely or profoundly handicapped.

e **False.** 1.5 per 1000, and increases with advancing maternal age.

Kendell, R.E. and Zealley, A.K. (eds.) (1993) *Companion to psychiatric studies*, 5th edn. Churchill Livingstone, Edinburgh, pp. 622–630.

5.9

a **True.** Language is a uniquely human ability, and Noam Chomsky argues that the grammar that allows us to acquire syntactic rules is innate—a genetic 'language acquisition device'—and independent of other cognitive processes.

b **True.** The deep structure of language is modified by transformational grammar, and Chomsky felt that all languages had commonalities at the deep syntactic level which facilitated childhood learning.

c **False.** Piaget thought that cognitive development was primary, in that it provides a capacity for symbol formation and rule manipulation upon which language is based.

d **False.** Freud thought that parapraxes, or 'slips of the tongue', represented a true but repressed intention. Word substitution errors are common in fluent aphasias, as seen in lesions to Wernicke's area.

e **False.** The Sapir–Whorf hypothesis (named after an American anthropologist and an insurance agent!) is a version of linguistic determinism and states that language determines the form of thought. Linguistic relativism states that different languages lead to different perceptions of the world.

Tantum, D. and Birchwood, M. (eds.) (1994) *Seminars in psychology and the social sciences*. Gaskell, London, pp. 68–76.

Questions
5.10

	[Certainty]		
Regarding the *t*-distribution	High	Med	Low
a It is a continuous probability distribution.	...	...	...
b It is used with large sample sizes.	...	...	...
c It is symmetrical about the mean.	...	...	...
d The tails are longer than in a normal distribution.	...	...	...
e It is named after its inventor, Joseph Teeson.	...	...	...

5.11

The rationale for systematic reviews include

	High	Med	Low
a Reducing large quantities of information into easily understood terms.	...	...	...
b Avoiding the need for further unnecessary work in the same field.	...	...	...
c To explain inconsistencies and conflicts in data.	...	...	...
d Increasing the power of studies by increasing sample size.	...	...	...
e Increasing precision in estimates of effect.	...	...	...

5.12

Factor analysis

	High	Med	Low
a Assumes that the relationship between variables and factors or dimensions is non-linear .	...	...	...
b Assumes that the variables are liable to random errors.	...	...	...
c Is used to establish if two variables vary in relation to each other.	...	...	...
d Was applied originally by psychologists.	...	...	...
e Includes the technique of principal factor analysis.	...	...	...

5.13

According to ICD 10, the following are true of Rett's syndrome:

	High	Med	Low
a Occurs more commonly in girls.	...	...	...
b Onset typically between 3 and 5 years of age.	...	...	...
c Stereotypies.	...	...	...
d Severe mental handicap.	...	...	...
e Seizures.	...	...	...

Answers
5.10

  a **True.** Like the normal distribution.
  b **False.** Usually under 30.
  c **True.**
  d **True.**
  e **False.**

Puri, B. and Tyrer, P. (1992) *Sciences basic to psychiatry*. Churchill Livingstone, Edinburgh, p. 227.

5.11

  a **True.**
  b **True.**
  c **True.**
  d **True.**
  e **True.**

Note: Systematic reviews are valuable techniques in research. They enable researchers, clinicians, and economists to make decisions about various diseases, outcomes, and treatment strategies by pooling data from similar lines of research which help establish whether findings are consistent and can be generalized across populations. The strict methods used in systematic reviews are to reduce bias and improve reliability and accuracy of conclusions.

Chalmers, I. and Altman, D.G. (eds.) (1995) *Systematic reviews*. BMJ Books, London, pp. 1–7.

5.12

  a **False.** The assumption is that relationships are linear.
  b **True.**
  c **False.** A correlation technique would be appropriate for this.
  d **True.**
  e **True.** Factor analysis is used to reduce the interrelationships within a large number of variables to a small number of statistically independent underlying factors or dimensions. These are related to the former variables in a linear manner.

Puri, B. and Tyrer, P. (1992) *Sciences basic to psychiatry*. Churchill Livingstone, Edinburgh, p. 250.

5.13

  a **False.** Has so far only been reported in girls.
  b **False.** Most cases have onset between 7 and 24 months.
  c **True.** Along with hyperventilation and loss of purposeful hand movements.
  d **True.** This is invariable.
  e **True.** Fits frequently develop during early or middle childhood.

World Health Organization (1992) *Tenth revision of the International Classification of Disease (ICD 10)*. WHO, Geneva. F84.2, p. 255.

Questions
5.14
	[Certainty]		
Antipsychotics that can be classed as atypical include	High	Med	Low
a Thioridazine.	...	...	...
b Sulpiride.	...	...	...
c Loxapine.	...	...	...
d Pimozide.	...	...	...
e Methaqualone.	...	...	...

5.15
With regard to cannabis:

a A withdrawal syndrome exists.	...	...	...
b Poor psychosocial out comes have been shown to result from regular use in adolescence.	...	...	...
c Chronic consumption generally leads to cognitive impairment.	...	...	...
d An increased risk of developing schizophrenia with prolonged heavy use has been shown.	...	...	...
e Structural brain abnormalities have been demonstrated in heavy chronic users.	...	...	...

5.16
The following should be avoided when taking phenelzine:

a Bananas.	...	...	...
b Avocados.	...	...	...
c Chianti.	...	...	...
d Cream cheese.	...	...	...
e Fresh liver.	...	...	...

Answers
5.14

a **True.** The term atypical strictly referred to the fact that the antipsychotic did not induce catalepsy in the rat, but now has been broadened to the properties of not provoking extrapyramidal side-effects (EPS) and not elevating serum prolactin. Thioridazine does have numerous potentially worrying side-effects.

b **True.** Sulpiride is a substituted benzamide acting primarily on D_2 receptors. EPS and galactorrhea have been associated with this compound, and hence the label 'atypical' is controversial.

c **True.** The only dibenzoxazepine commercially available, and the molecule is similar to the tricyclic dibenzodiazepines such as clozapine except for an oxygen for nitrogen substitution in the central ring.

d **False.** This drug has a long half life and tendency to lead to arrythmias (annual ECG recommended). Said to be particularly suitable for monosymptomatic delusional states.

e **False.** This is an obsolete barbiturate.

Note: The term 'atypical' is seemingly being applied to antipsychotics with increasing imprecision, but the area remains fashionable. Other 'atypicals' are clozapine, risperidone, sertindole, olanzapine, quetiapine, and the now withdrawn remoxipride.

Kerwin, R.W. (1994) The new atypical antipsychotics: a lack of extrapyramidal side-effects and new routes in schizophrenia research. *British Journal of Psychiatry* 164, 141–148.

British National Formulary, Section 4.2.

5.15

a **True.** Although generally mild and thus not often reported as such.

b **True.**

c **False.** However, research is of low quality. Some impairment of task performance for selective attention; visual and spatial memory; and visuomotor function has been documented

d **True.** Although this is a controversial area.

e **False.**

Hall, W. and Solowij, N. (1997) Long term cannabis use and mental health. *British Journal of Psychiatry* 171, 107–108.

5.16

a **False.** But banana skins should be avoided.

b **True.**

c **True.**

d **False.** All cheese except cream and cottage cheese.

e **True.** Fresh meat is acceptable but not offal.

Note: Tyramine-rich foods inhibit the peripheral metabolism of pressor amines, in the presence of an monoamine oxidase inhibitor (MAOI). Even the reversible inhibitors of monoamine oxidase (RIMAs) (e.g. moclobemide) are not absolutely safe.

Puri, B. (1995) *Saunders' pocket essentials of psychiatry*. Saunders, Philadelphia, pp. 99–100.

Questions

5.17

	[Certainty]		
In genetic research	High	Med	Low
a Mendel's first law describes separation of paired alleles.	...	...	...
b Mendel's second law states that there is independent assortment of different alleles.	...	...	...
c Acute intermittent porphyria (AIP) is an example of autosomal dominant inheritance with complete penetrance.	...	...	...
d The heritability of a trait is the proportion of the phenotypic variance of the trait that is contributed by the genetic component.	...	...	...
e X-linked disorders affect only male children.	...	...	...

5.18

The following neurotransmitters inhibit feeding:			
a Galanin.	...	...	...
b Noradrenaline.	...	...	...
c Cholecystikinin (CCK).	...	...	...
d Serotonin.	...	...	...
e Neuropeptide Y.	...	...	...

5.19

Regarding the scalp EEG:			
a The international 10–20 system of positioning is standard.	...	...	...
b It is unavailable in ambulatory form.	...	...	...
c β rhythm disappears when the eyes are open.	...	...	...
d θ waves vary between 4 and 8 Hz.	...	...	...
e High amplitude δ activity is common in the awake adult.	...	...	...

Answers
5.17

a **True.** This is also known as the law of segregation.

b **True.**

c **False.** AIP is the most common type of porphyria in the UK population. It is autosomal dominant but exhibits only incomplete penetrance.

d **True.**

e **False.** X-linked dominant disorders are thought to exist, e.g. Rett's syndrome, and so females could be affected. Also rarely a female child of parents who both have an abnormal gene on their X chromosome could suffer from an X-linked recessive disorder.

Puri, B. and Tyrer, P. (1992) *Sciences basic to psychiatry*. Churchill Livingstone, Edinburgh, pp. 153–159.

5.18

a **False.** Along with the opioids and growth-hormone releasing factor, galanin stimulates feeding. Neurotransmitters that increase feeding when injected into the hypothalamus also increase gastric acidity, and decrease other behaviours such as grooming and sexual activity.

b **False.**

c **True.** The first satiety transmitter discovered. Also present in the gut where it regulates postprandial bile release. There are two CCK receptors, with CCKA regulating appetite, feeding and possibly pain, and CCKB having some influence over emotion.

d **True.** A common side-effect of SSRI antidepressants, and fluoxetine is licensed for the treatment of bulimia.

e **False.** Neuropeptide Y is the most potent appetite-stimulant transmitter discovered. It is also a powerful vasoconstrictor. An effective antagonist would have enormous clinical (and commercial) value.

Morgan, G. and Butler, S. (eds.) (1993) *Seminars in basic neurosciences*. Gaskell, London, pp. 236–237.

5.19

a **True.** Electrodes are positioned at defined places.

b **False.** There is a format analogous to the 24-hour ECG, which is recorded on cassette tape.

c **False.** α rhythm disappears.

d **True.**

e **False.** High amplitude θ and δ activity do not occur in the awake adult.

Puri, B. and Tyrer, P. (1992) *Sciences basic to psychiatry*. Churchill Livingstone, Edinburgh, pp. 62–64.

Questions

5.20

	[Certainty]		
Physiological correlates of rapid eye movement (REM) sleep include:	High	Med	Low
a Decreased recall of dreaming if awoken from REM sleep.	...	...	...
b Decreased complexity of dreams.	...	...	...
c Decreased parasympathetic activity.	...	...	...
d Increased vaginal blood flow.	...	...	...
e Myoclonic jerks.	...	...	...

5.21

The following statements are true:
a Bombesin is a neuropeptide.
b Cholecystikinin coexists with GABA in the cerebral cortex.
c Corticotrophin releasing factor output is reduced during stress.
d Intravenous cholecystokinin has proved effective in reducing the binge eating associated with bulimia nervosa.
e Corticotrophin-related peptides have been shown to enhance attention.

5.22

Regarding group processes and non-verbal communication:
a A 'shift to risk' describes an individual's likelihood of decision about his or her future after discussion within a group setting.
b In large group settings centralized networks are highly efficient in dealing with complex problems.
c People with anxiety and alcohol problems look at their interviewer less than controls.
d The family is an example of a primary group.
e Group cohesiveness is unrelated to hostility to other groups.

5.23

The following are correct pairings:
a Mechanic—suicide.
b Durkheim—illness behaviour.
c Goffman—total institution.
d Barton—institutional neurosis.
e Parsons—sick role.

Answers

5.20

a **False.** Increased recall of dreaming if awoken from REM sleep.

b **False.** Increased complexity of dreams.

c **False.** Increased parasympathetic activity, including increased heart rate, elevation of blood pressure, and increased respiratory rate.

d **True.**

e **True.**

Puri, B. and Hall, A.D. (1998) *Revision notes in psychiatry* 13. Arnold, London, p. 143.

5.21

a **True.** Found in the central nervous system, gastrointestinal tract and lungs.

b **True.** Along with dopamine in the mesencephalon, and 5HT in the medulla.

c **False.** The hypothalamic–pituitary–suprarenal cortex axis is involved in the endocrine response to stress.

d **False.** Although it does inhibit feeding.

e **True.** Although studies on the effects of cognitive functioning in the elderly are not consistently positive.

Puri, B. and Tyrer, P. (1992) *Sciences basic to psychiatry*. Churchill Livingstone, Edinburgh, pp. 45–46.

5.22

a **True.** Individuals are more likely to take risky decisions about themselves than groups.

b **False.** In a large group settings centralized networks are highly efficient in dealing with simple problems and become inefficient in dealing with complex problems.

c **False.** People with schizophrenia and depression look at their interviewer less than controls.

d **True.** In which interpersonal relationships take place on a frequent face-to-face basis.

e **False.** It is related.

Weller, M. and Eysenck, M. (1991) *The Scientific Basis of Psychiatry*, 2nd edn. Saunders, Philadelphia, pp. 461–467.

5.23

a **False.** Mechanic—illness behaviour.

b **False.** Durkheim—suicide.

c **True.** Examples of total institutions are the older asylums, prisons, and monasteries.

d **True.** The apathetic, passive, withdrawn state of persons living in total institutions.

e **True.** The role given by society to a sick person.

Puri, B. and Tyrer, P. (1992) *Sciences basic to psychiatry*. Churchill Livingstone, Edinburgh, pp. 294–296.

Questions

5.24

	[Certainty]		
According to Zola, triggers for seeking medical care are	High	Med	Low
a Perceived interference with personal relations.	...	...	...
b Pressure from others.	...	...	...
c The occurrence of an interpersonal crisis.	...	...	...
d Perceived interference with vocational or physical activity.	...	...	...
e Temporalizing of symptomatology.	...	...	...

5.25

According to Parsons' theory of the 'sick role'			
a A doctor is obliged to treat the patient's illness.	...	...	...
b The individual has the right to exemption from blame for the illness.	...	...	...
c The individual is obliged to want to recover.	...	...	...
d The individual has the right to refuse treatment for the condition.	...	...	...
e The doctor is able to define and legitimize the illness.	...	...	...

Clinical

5.26

Poor outcome in affective disorder is predicted by			
a A positive family history of depressive disorder.	...	...	...
b Comorbid dysthymia.	...	...	...
c Severity of initial psychopathology.	...	...	...
d Late but insidious onset.	...	...	...
e Reduced perfusion of the dorsolateral prefrontal cortex seen by functional neuroimaging techniques.	...	...	...

Answers
5.24

   a **True.**
   b **True.**
   c **True.**
   d **True.**
   e **True.** i.e. setting a deadline for the disappearance of symptoms after which help will be sought

Patrick, D.L. and Scambler, G. (1982) *Sociology as applied to medicine.* Baillière Tindall, London, pp. 49–50.

5.25

   a **False.**
   b **True.**
   c **True.**
   d **False.**
   e **True.**

Note: Parsons describes two 'rights' of sick individuals—exemption from blame for the illness, and exemption from duties and responsibilities such as work. He also describes two 'obligations' of sick individuals—to want to recover and to accept appropriate help.

Puri, B. and Tyrer, P. (1992) *Sciences basic to psychiatry.* Churchill Livingstone, Edinburgh, p. 294.

Clinical

5.26

   a **False.** Positive family history is linked to poor prognosis in schizophrenia, not depression.
   b **True.** So-called 'double depression'.
   c **True.** In the 18-year follow-up conducted by Lee and Murray (1988), the long term outcome of affective disorder was generally bad—25% were dead or had continuing disability.
   d **False.** Early onset is predictive. An early, insidious onset is worse in schizophrenia.
   e **False.** This, along with reduced perfusion in the cingulate gyrus and left angular cortex, was the 'anatomy of melancholia' described using positron emission tomography (PET).

Buckey P.F., Bird, J., and Harrison, G. (1995) *Examination notes in psychiatry,* (3rd edn. Butterworth-Heinemann, Oxford, pp. 51–55.

Lee, A.S. and Murray, R.M. (1988) The long-term outcome of Maudsley depressives. *Brit. J. Psych,* 153, pp. 741–751.

Questions

5.27

[Certainty]

With regard to postnatal illness:

	High	Med	Low

a A positive association has been found between postnatal
   depression and being unmarried.   ...   .

b Studies have shown that women said to be 'emotionally
   unstable' in the first week after childbirth are at
   increased risk of subsequent depression.   ...   .

c Puerperal psychoses are more likely after second and
   subsequent births.   ...   .

d Mothers with previous histories of bipolar illness or
   puerperal psychosis have a 1 in 8 risk of an affective
   illness after childbirth.   ...   .

e Postnatal blues are not linked with more serious
   psychiatric disorders.   ...   .

5.28

Long-term outcome in schizophrenia

a Is more favourable now than it was in the first three
   decades of this century.   ...   .

b Is more favourable in developed countries.   ...   .

c Is less favourable if perplexity is present at the onset of
   the disease.   ...   .

d Is more favourable if there are few abnormal premorbid
   personality traits present.   ...   .

e Is more favourable if there is a family history of
   depressive illness.   ...   .

5.29

The following are recognized in schizophrenia:

a Fathers of schizophrenics being from the same social
   class as the general population.   ...   .

b Reduced ventricle to brain ratios.   ...   .

c Increased redundancy of speech.   ...   .

d Increased schizophrenic spectrum disorder in relatives.   ...   .

e A higher incidence in second generation Afro-Caribbean
   populations in the UK compared with first generation
   populations.   ...   .

Answers

5.27

a **False.** No association has been found.

b **True.**

c **True.** Other risk factors include being unmarried, perinatal death, and delivery by caesarean section.

d **False.** 1 in 2 to 1 in 4.

e **False.** Research has shown that severe postnatal blues may be linked to more serious psychiatric disorder.

Gelder, M., Gath, D., Mayou, R., and Cowen, P. (eds.) (1996) *The Oxford textbook of psychiatry*, 3rd edn. Oxford University Press, Oxford, pp. 395–397.

Kendell, R.E. and Zealley, A.K. (eds.) (1993) *Companion to psychiatric studies*, 5th edn. Churchill Livingstone, Edinburgh, pp. 579–583.

5.28

a **True.**

b **False.** A finding of the International Pilot Study in Schizophrenia was that the prognosis was more favourable in 'developing' countries.

c **False.** More favourable.

d **True.**

e **True.**

Note: Features at onset of the illness and premorbid personality traits appear to be the most useful indicators of prognosis.

Kendell, R.E. and Zealley, A.K. (eds.) (1993) *Companion to psychiatric studies*, 5th edn. Churchill Livingstone, Edinburgh, pp. 414–417.

5.29

a **True.** Patients with schizophrenia are not, in keeping with the theory of social drift.

b **False.** Increased ventricle to brain ratios.

c **False.** Their speech is less redundant, i.e. if every fourth or fifth word is missing a reader with no prior knowledge would be less successful at guessing the missing words.

d **True.**

e **True.**

Kendell, R.E. and Zealley, A.K. (eds.) (1993) *Companion to psychiatric studies*, 5th edn. Churchill Livingstone, Edinburgh, pp. 397–423.

Questions

5.30

[Certainty]

The following statements regarding alcohol consumption are true:

	High	Med	Low
a Increased advertising and marketing has been shown to be linked to increased alcohol consumption in Britain.	...	...	...
b Patterns of alcohol consumption throughout Britain are similar.	...	...	...
c The greatest proportion of alcohol related harm in a society is attributable to very heavy drinkers.	...	...	...
d Coronary artery disease protection by light alcohol consumption is probably mediated by HDL-cholesterol levels.	...	...	...
e The prevalence of alcoholism in a population increases with age.	...	...	...

5.31

Notification is required by law for dependence on

a Pethidine.	...	...	...
b LSD.	...	...	...
c Barbiturates.	...	...	...
d Cocaine.	...	...	...
e Ecstasy.	...	...	...

5.32

The following help differentiate between dementia and pseudodementia:

a Effort at task performance.	...	...	...
b Mini-mental state examination test score.	...	...	...
c Single photon emission tomography (SPET/SPECT) scanning.	...	...	...
d Positive family history of dementia.	...	...	...
e Extent to which the patient complains of their problems.	...	...	...

Answers
5.30

   a **True.** As does increasing the number of outlets, extension of licensing hours, and falling relative price of alcohol.

   b **False.** Although the mean consumption is similar in England, Wales, and Scotland, Scottish adult males tend to drink in 'binges'.

   c **False.** Moderately heavy drinkers because there are many more of them.

   d **True.** Light = 1–3 units per day.

   e **False.** Surveys record low rates of drinking problems after the age of 50.

Kendell, R.E. and Zealley, A.K. (eds.) (1993) *Companion to psychiatric studies*, 5th edn. Churchill Livingstone, Edinburgh, pp. 361–365.

5.31

   a **True.** If drug addiction is suspected the Chief Medical Officer must be notified. Diamorphine (heroin), dipipanone, methadone, morphine, opium, and phenazocine are also drugs that are notifiable.

   b **False.**

   c **False.**

   d **True.**

   e **False.** Class A drugs include cocaine, LSD, heroin, morphine, methadone, pethidine, opium, as well as Class B drugs when prepared for injection (e.g. amphetamines).

Chick, J. and Cantwell, R. (eds.) (1994) *Seminars in alcohol and drug misuse*. Gaskell, London, p. 36.

5.32

   a **True.** Task performance is poor in pseudodementia, whereas the demented patient struggles for the answer.

   b **False.** Islands of normality and specific memory gaps are more common in pseudodementia, but the total MMSE score may be unrevealing.

   c **True.** Parietotemporal and frontal deficits are common in dementia, but cerebral blood flow is normal or only reduced in the left hemisphere in those with pseudodementia.

   d **False.** A positive family history for affective disorder, and a previous history of depression make depressive pseudodementia more likely.

   e **True.** An exaggerated presentation of symptoms is seen in depressive pseudo-dementia, whereas those with dementia tend to conceal their disabilities. Other clues to pseudodementia are an underlying low mood, a tendency to reply 'I don't know', and a clear onset.

Puri, B.K. (1995) *Saunder's pocket essentials of psychiatry*. Saunders, Philadelphia, pp. 82–83.

Questions

5.33

In epilepsy

[Certainty]

High   Med   Low

a A temporal lobe behavioural syndrome is described
which includes hyperemotionality and hyposexuality.

b In male epileptics who are on treatment, free testosterone
levels tend to be low.

c Violent offences have been found to be 40% higher
among epileptics compared with other offenders.

d The interictal psychoses occur in the setting of a
decreased conscious level.

e About 15% of those with temporal lobe epilepsy may go
on to develop a chronic schizophrenia like psychosis.

5.34

In a patient presenting with hypertonia, pyrexia, and
autonomic lability, the following are a likely underlying cause:

a A brain stem haemorrhage.

b Catatonia.

c Acquired immunodeficiency syndrome.

d Meningitis.

e Shy–Drager syndrome.

5.35

Pseudobulbar palsy

a Can be caused by cerebrovascular disease.

b Causes dysphagia.

c Inhibits the jaw jerk.

d Produces muscular atrophy.

e Can lead to emotional lability.

Answers
5.33

    a **True.** Due to limbic system kindling.

    b **True.** Liver enzyme induction by anticonvulsants.

    c **False.** Although prevalence of epilepsy among male prisoners is 3 times higher than the general population.

    d **False.** Clear consciousness.

    e **False.** About 2%, after an average of 7 years of seizures.

Kendell, R.E. and Zealley, A.K. (eds.) (1993) *Companion to psychiatric studies*, 5th edn. Churchill Livingstone, Edinburgh, pp. 349–355.

5.34

    a **True.** A fever can accompany the early stages of a 'locked in' syndrome.

    b **False.** Catatonic symptoms seem to be gradually disappearing. Although stereotypy, the 'psychological pillow,' and waxy flexibility consist of increased muscular tone, catatonic signs are usually said to be those of excessive or automatic obedience (e.g. *mitgehen*). The temperature and cardiovascular system should be normal.

    c **True.** There are protean CNS manifestations of AIDS.

    d **True.** As well as encephalitis.

    e **False.** This is a multisystem atrophy, akin to Parkinson's disease, characterized by autonomic failure but not by pyrexia.

Note: In a psychotic patient with these symptoms the most likely diagnosis is the neuroleptic malignant syndrome. The differential diagnosis and management of this condition is a favourite exam topic.

Gelder, M., Gath, D., Mayou, R., and Cowen, P. (eds.) (1996) *The Oxford textbook of psychiatry*, 3rd edn. Oxford University Press, Oxford, pp. 554–555

5.35

    a **True.** Pseudobulbar palsy can be due to motor neurone or cerebrovascular disease, as well as multiple sclerosis.

    b **True.** There is apparent weakness of the muscles of mastication and expression, leading to difficulty in chewing and an expressionless face.

    c **False.** The jaw jerk is exaggerated, the tongue immobile.

    d **False.** Atrophy is more usually associated with lower motor neurone loss.

    e **True.**

Souhami, R.L. and Moxham, J. (eds.) (1990) *Textbook of medicine*. Churchill Livingstone, Edinburgh, p. 898.

Questions
5.36

	[Certainty]		
Non-epileptic or pseudoseizures	High	Med	Low
a Are rarely seen in true epilepsy.	...	...	...
b Give rise to a markedly elevated serum prolactin.	...	...	...
c Can be consciously provoked.	...	...	...
d Are often diagnosed using video telemetry.	...	...	...
e Are usually due to a histrionic personality disorder.	...	...	...

5.37

Correct associations include			
a Collective unconscious—Adler.	...	...	...
b Masculine protest—Jung.	...	...	...
c Oedipal conflict—Sigmund Freud.	...	...	...
d Id psychology—Bowlby.	...	...	...
e Maternal deprivation—Klein.	...	...	...

5.38

The following are necessary for supportive (level 1) psychotherapy:

a Understanding of problems in psychological terms.	...	...	...
b Patient's motivation for insight and change.	...	...	...
c Ego strength.	...	...	...
d Capacity to form and sustain relationships.	...	...	...
e Lack of impulsivity.	...	...	...

5.39

The following are associated with Winnicott:			
a The collective unconscious.	...	...	...
b Transitional phenomenon.	...	...	...
c The 'good enough mother'.	...	...	...
d Cannibalistic monsters.	...	...	...
e The paranoid–schizoid position.	...	...	...

Answers
5.36

a **False.** Pseudoseizures, or non-epileptic seizures, can be notoriously difficult to diagnose.

b **False.** Only elevated after a true seizure.

c **True.**

d **True.** Simultaneous 24 hour video and EEG monitoring.

e **False.** Causation is multifactorial, but sometimes is linked to childhood abuse and personality disturbance.

Fenwick, P. (1995) Psychiatric disorder and epilepsy. In *Epilepsy*, 2nd edn., ed. A. Hopkins, S. Shorvon, and G. Cascino. Chapman & Hall, London, pp. 451–498.

Kendell, R.E. and Zealley, A.K. (eds.) (1993) *Companion to psychiatric studies*, 5th edn. Churchill Livingstone, Edinburgh, pp. 352–353.

5.37

a **False.** Collective unconscious—Jung.

b **False.** Masculine protest—Adler.

c **True.**

d **False.** Id psychology—Klein.

e **False.** Maternal deprivation—Bowlby.

Brown, D. and Pedder, J. (1991) *Introduction to psychotherapy*, 2nd edn. Routledge, London, pp. 101–106.

5.38

a **False.**

b **False.**

c **False.**

d **False.**

e **False.**

Note: These are selection criteria for exploratory (level 3) psychotherapy.

Brown, D. and Pedder, J. (1991) *Introduction to psychotherapy*, 2nd edn. Routledge, London, pp. 180–186.

5.39

a **False.** The collective unconscious is associated with Carl Gustav Jung.

b **True.** Designating intermediate areas of experience, e.g. between the thumb and the teddy bear, or oral eroticism and true object relations.

c **True.** The necessity of a degree of 'maternal preoccupation'.

d **False.**

e **False.** The paranoid–schizoid position is associated with Melanie Klein.

Brown, D. and Pedder, J. (1991) *Introduction to psychotherapy*, 2nd edn. Routledge, London, pp. 106–107.

Questions
5.40

	[Certainty]		
Following bereavement, factors predicting a pathological grief reaction include:	High	Med	Low
a Previous depressive illness.	...	...	...
b Early parental loss.	...	...	...
c A narcissistic relationship with the deceased.	...	...	...
d Alcohol dependence.	...	...	...
e Not being able to see the body of the deceased.	...	...	...

5.41

The following help distinguish Asperger's syndrome from infantile autism:

	High	Med	Low
a Clumsiness.	...	...	...
b A relatively low performance compared to verbal IQ.	...	...	...
c Speech disorder.	...	...	...
d Right hemisphere deficits.	...	...	...
e Relative prevalence.	...	...	...

5.42

Specific reading retardation (SRR)

	High	Med	Low
a Has a prevalence of 1% in inner city 10 year olds.	...	...	...
b Has equal prevalence in boys and girls.	...	...	...
c Has a good social prognosis.	...	...	...
d Is associated with normal language development.	...	...	...
e Is also known as dyslexia.	...	...	...

Answers
5.40

a **True.** Several authors, including Murray Parkes, have found a pre-existing low self-esteem and tendency to self-blame is predictive.

b **True.** Compare with Brown and Harris's vulnerability factors for depression.

c **True.** As well as a dependent or ambivalent relationship.

d **False.** No evidence for this, but a lack of social support is predictive.

e **True.** Any uncertain death, where the body is missing or mutilated beyond recognition.

Zisook, S. (ed.) (1987) *Psychiatric Clinics of North America* 10(3), 487–499.

5.41

a **True.** This is said to be a defining feature of Asperger's, along with idiosyncratic interests and a reasonably preserved IQ.

b **True.** In autism the performance IQ is usually higher than the verbal IQ, which is the reverse of Asperger's.

c **True.** Asperger's sufferers are meant to be fluent but original language users, whereas autistics often have a severe expressive speech disorder with poor prosody.

d **True.** Asperger's has been associated with aminoacidurias and other CNS disorders. The deficits are said to be consistent with right hemisphere lesions.

e **True.** Asperger's is a rare disorder principally affecting boys (7 : 1).

World Health Organization (1992). *Tenth revision of the International Classification of Disease (ICD 10)*. WHO, Geneva, pp. 258–259.

5.42

a **False.** 10%.

b **False.** It is three times more common in boys than girls.

c **False.** One third of those with SRR have a conduct disorder and the prognosis socially is not good.

d **False.** It is associated with delay in speaking.

e **True.**

Black, D. and Cottrell, D. (eds.) (1993) *Seminars in child and adolescent psychiatry*. Gaskell, London, pp. 16–17.

Questions

5.43

	[Certainty]		
The following are examples of dissociation:	High	Med	Low
a Fugue.	...	...	...
b Derealization.	...	...	...
c Trance.	...	...	...
d Multiple personality.	...	...	...
e Somnambulism.	...	...	...

5.44

In the study of anxiety disorders			
a Abnormalities in brain structure have been found in those with panic disorder.	...	...	...
b Ritanserin has anti-panic effects.	...	...	...
c Abnormalities of melatonin production are common in panic patients.	...	...	...
d Panic disorder patients tend to interpret bodily sensations in a catastrophic manner.	...	...	...
e Abnormality of the GABA system is a feature of panic disorder.	...	...	...

5.45

The following preclude the accused from standing trial:			
a Being disorientated in time.	...	...	...
b Inability to instruct counsel.	...	...	...
c Believing the judge is an impostor.	...	...	...
d Not understanding the legal process.	...	...	...
e Being mentally impaired.	...	...	...

Answers
5.43

a **True.** Fugue means flight, and a dissociative fugue has the features of dissociative amnesia in the context of organized travel, usually with self-care maintained.

b **False.** A neurotic disorder in which the sufferer feels unreal, remote, or automatized. Insight is retained.

c **True.** Trance disorders are involuntary and intrude into ordinary activities. There is temporary loss of both personal identity and awareness of surroundings.

d **True.** A less common dissociative disorder, like Ganser's syndrome. Usually there are two personalities, with one dominant. Switch between the personalities is precipitated by trauma.

e **False.** Sleepwalking is probably an arousal disorder, particularly from deep sleep. There are many clinical and pathogenetic similarities to sleep (night) terrors.

World Health Organization (1992) *Tenth revision of the International Classification of Disease (ICD 10)*. WHO, Geneva, pp. 151–161.

5.44

a **True.** Abnormalities in the right parahippocampal area.

b **False.** It may exacerbate anxiety as it is a 5HT antagonist.

c **True.** There is increased nocturnal production.

d **True.** Hence may respond to cognitive therapies.

e **True.** Along with abnormalities of 5HT and noradrenaline.

Gelder, M., Gath, D., Mayou, R., and Cowen, P. (eds.) (1996) *The Oxford textbook of psychiatry*, 3rd edn. Oxford University Press, Oxford, pp. 176–179.

Kendell, R.E. and Zealley, A.K. (eds.) (1993) *Companion to psychiatric studies*, 5th edn. Churchill Livingstone, Edinburgh, pp. 495–498.

5.45

a **False.** Many 'normal' people are.

b **True.** Being sane and fit to plead includes this, as well as understanding the difference between guilty and not guilty; and the process and consequences of legal action.

c **False.** Unless the accused is thought to be insane in bar of trial by the independent psychiatrist, because of a floridly active severe psychosis.

d **True.** See above.

e **False.** Not automatically, but having a learning disability can lead to being declared 'unfit to plead'. If there is doubt, the accused can be re-examined on the morning of the trial.

Kendell, R.E. and Zealley, A.K. (eds.) (1993) *Companion to psychiatric studies*, 5th edn. Churchill Livingstone, Edinburgh, pp. 809–811.

Questions

5.46

[Certainty]

The following statements are true:

		High	Med	Low
a	Approximately 50% of hospital orders are created along with restrictions on discharge.	...	...	...
b	Restricted patients may never be discharged or transferred without permission from the Home/Scottish Office.	...	...	...
c	The Butler Committee was responsible for the setting up of an advisory board on restricted patients.	...	...	...
d	The use of the interim Hospital Order may be particularly useful for those with psychopathic personality disorder.	...	...	...
e	A psychiatric in-patient is ineligible to vote.	...	...	...

5.47

The following are useful in the management of treatment-resistant schizophrenia:

		High	Med	Low
a	Sodium valproate.	...	...	...
b	Cognitive therapy.	...	...	...
c	Tertiary referral centres.	...	...	...
d	Narcotherapy.	...	...	...
e	Insight-orientated psychotherapy.	...	...	...

5.48

Lithium carbonate should be avoided in

		High	Med	Low
a	Liver disease.	...	...	...
b	Moderate renal failure.	...	...	...
c	Combination with L-tryptophan.	...	...	...
d	Pregnancy.	...	...	...
e	Combination with a thiazide diuretic.	...	...	...

5.49

Cardiac complications of anorexia nervosa include:

		High	Med	Low
a	Reduction of the corrected QT interval.	...	...	...
b	Tachycardia.	...	...	...
c	A decrease in cardiac size.	...	...	...
d	Hypotension.	...	...	...
e	Mitral valve prolapse.	...	...	...

Answers
5.46

  a **False.** Around 15%.
  b **True.**
  c **False.** The Aarvold Committee (1973).
  d **True.**
  e **False.** Those who are compulsorily detained may not register for the electoral roll.

Kendell, R.E. and Zealley, A.K. (eds.) (1993) *Companion to psychiatric studies*, 5th edn. Churchill Livingstone, Edinburgh, pp. 796, 797, 800.

5.47

  a **True.** Both as adjunctive therapy, and to counteract the proconvulsant effects of high dose clozapine.
  b **True.** Approximately 30% of resistant delusions can respond to specialized cognitive therapy.
  c **False.** These exist, but there are no controlled data to suggest outcome is improved.
  d **False.**
  e **False.** Most dynamic therapists and analysts feel psychosis is a contra-indication to dynamic psychotherapy.

Johnstone, E. C and Sandler, R. (1996) Treatment resistance in schizophrenia (editorial). *British Medical Journal* 312 (7027), 325–326.

5.48

  a **False.** Lithium is eliminated by the kidneys.
  b **True.**
  c **False.** This is often a useful combination in treatment resistant depression.
  d **True.** Due to teratogenic effects.
  e **True.** As it can lead to lithium toxicity. Close monitoring is recommended.

British National Formulary, Section 4.2.3.

5.49

  a **False.** Prolongation of the corrected QT interval may lead to fatal arrythmias.
  b **False.** Bradycardia is typical.
  c **True.**
  d **True.**
  e **True.**

Beaumont, P.J., Russell, J.D., Touyz, S.W. (1993) Treatment of anorexia nervosa. *Lancet* 34, 1635–1640.

Kendell, R.E. and Zealley, A.K. (eds.) (1993) *Companion to psychiatric studies*, 5th edn. Churchill Livingstone, Edinburgh, pp. 526–529

Questions

5.50

[Certainty]

In Down's syndrome	High	Med	Low
a Increased paternal age is a relative risk factor.	...	...	...
b Only a minority of sufferers have an IQ greater than 50.	...	...	...
c In translocation cases the patient has 47 chromosomes.	...	...	...
d Hypothyroidism is commonly seen.	...	...	...
e Those with dementia have an increased P300 latency on evoked potential studies.	...	...	...

Answers
5.50

    a **True.** Increased maternal age is a well known risk factor, for mothers aged 45 or over the incidence is 1 in 50. However, increased paternal age and X-ray radiation have also been implicated.

    b **True.** Among patients with an IQ less than 50, one-third have Down's syndrome.

    c **False.** In translocation, the carriers have only 45 chromosomes, whereas the patient has 46 and may manifest all or a few features of Down's syndrome. Translocation accounts for about 4% of all cases.

    d **True.** Hypothyroidism and the cognitive decline usually begin in middle age.

    e **True.** Cortical senile plaques are evident early in life, probably due to genetic programming, but clinical dementia occurs later. The increase in P300 latency is evident around 37 years of age, and has been shown to be present in all of a sample of Down's syndrome patient with early dementia.

Kendell, R.E. and Zealley, A.K. (eds.) (1993) *Companion to psychiatric studies*, 5th edn. Churchill Livingstone, Edinburgh, pp. 629–30.

Paper 6: Questions

Basic science

6.1

	[Certainty]		
The cerebellum	High	Med	Low
a Receives mossy fibres as its sole major input pathway.	...	...	...
b Is the only area of the nervous system to cross the midline uninterrupted.	...	...	...
c Contains excitatory interneurons called basket cells and stellate cells.	...	...	...
d Has outputs to the thalamus and motor cortex.	...	...	...
e Literally means 'little brain'.	...	...	...

6.2

Cerebrospinal fluid (CSF)

a Is located in the subarachnoid space. ... ...

b Is formed by a passive process. ... ...

c Is re-absorbed via an active process. ... ...

d Total volume is approximately 100 ml in healthy subjects. ... ...

e Passes from the fourth ventricle through the foraminae of Magendie and Luschka. ... ...

6.3

Pick's disease

a Shows marked frontal and anterior temporal lobe atrophy. ... ...

b Is familial in 1 in 20 cases. ... ...

c Affects men twice as frequently as women. ... ...

d Is microscopically characterized by 'balloon cells'. ... ...

e Is not associated with nerve cell gliosis. ... ...

Paper 6: Answers

Basic science

6.1

a **False.** Mossy fibres and climbing fibres comprise the inputs to the cerebellar cortex. An output is generated, in turn, to the cerebellar nuclei via Purkinje neurons. Mossy fibres originate from many areas including the vestibular labyrinth and sensory cortex. Climbing fibres come from the inferior olive.

b **True.** The human cerebellum has similar wiring to lower vertebrates, but is substantially larger.

c **False.** The inhibitory interneurons are the Golgi cells, basket cells, and stellate cells. Excitatory granule cells are the intrinsic neurons linking the mossy fibres to the Purkinje cell pathways.

d **True.** There are outputs to the vestibular nucleus, red nucleus, thalamus, and motor cortex.

e **True.** The cerebellum provides information about movements over the whole body, and provides cortical feedback on motor activity allowing coordination.

Morgan, G. and Butler, S. (eds.) (1993) *Seminars in basic neurosciences.* Gaskell, London, pp. 60–61.

6.2

a **True.**

b **False.** An active process by the ependymal lining of the choroid plexuses of the lateral, third, and fourth ventricles.

c **False.** A passive process by the arachnoid villi of the dural venous sinuses.

d **False.** Approximately 140 ml.

e **True.**

Puri, B. and Tyrer, P. (1992) *Sciences basic to psychiatry.* Churchill Livingstone, Edinburgh, pp. 21–22.

6.3

a **True.** A degree of general atrophy is also seen.

b **False.** 1 in 10.

c **False.** Twice as frequently seen in women.

d **True.** They are not a constant feature, but characteristic.

e **False.** There is fibrous gliosis in cortex and underlying white matter.

Note: Onset is in the 5th decade. Macroscopically the 'knife-edge gyri' of the often dramatic atrophy is seen. Microscopically there is nerve cell loss and gliosis, as well as swollen Pick cells and Pick inclusion bodies. These Pick bodies stain like Alzheimer tangles but lack paired helical filaments.

Lishman, W.A. (1998) *Organic psychiatry*, 3rd edn. Blackwell Science, Oxford, pp. 460–462.

Questions
6.4

[Certainty]

Prion protein	High	Med	Low
a Is a normal brain protein.	...	...	...
b In the soluble form is responsible for spongiform changes and cell death.	...	...	...
c In the insoluble form is resistant to the actions of proteases.	...	...	...
d Is demonstrated in the brains of subjects with spongiform changes.	...	...	...
e Is transmissible by oral ingestion.	...	...	...

6.5

Concerning the neurobiology of schizophrenia:

	High	Med	Low
a There is an increased P300 latency in many cases.	...	...	...
b Those affected and their first degree relatives display eye-tracking abnormalities.	...	...	...
c An increased incidence of non-localizing neurological signs has been found in schizophrenia.	...	...	...
d There are enlarged lateral ventricles in all cases.	...	...	...
e Increased cerebral activity in the frontal lobes has been found in many cases.	...	...	...

6.6

The following are autosomal recessive disorders of carbohydrate and lipid metabolism:

	High	Med	Low
a Pompe's disease.	...	...	...
b Type II tyrosinaemia.	...	...	...
c Hurler's syndrome.	...	...	...
d Hyperuricaemia.	...	...	...
e Tuberous sclerosis.	...	...	...

Answers
6.4

a **True.** However, prion diseases occur when the normal soluble form (PrP^C) undergoes a conformational change to the insoluble form(PrP^{Sc}).

b **False.** See above. The soluble form can transform to the insoluble form spontaneously. This is thought to be the case in Creutzfeldt–Jacob disease (CJD).

c **True.**

d **True.**

e **True.** Prion diseases are thought to include Kuru (associated with cannibalism), scrapie, bovine spongiform encephalitis (BSE), CJD, and new variant CJD.

Fleminger, S. and Curtis, D. (1997) Prion diseases. *British Journal of Psychiatry* 170, 103–105.

Lishman, W.A. (1998) *Organic psychiatry*, 3rd edn. Blackwell Science, Oxford, pp. 474–476.

6.5

a **True.** P300 is a cognitive event-related potential which has been shown to have reduced amplitude and prolonged latency in schizophrenics and some of their relatives.

b **True.**

c **True.** Many authors now view a proportion of cases as neurodevelopmental in origin, with delayed milestones and later cognitive and cerebral disturbances. Males may be more susceptible to the postulated prenatal and perinatal insults.

d **False.** Lateral and third ventriculomegaly is seen in many but not all cases.

e **False.** A 'hypofrontality' theory of schizophrenia has been proposed.

Gelder, M., Gath, D., Mayou, R., and Cowen, P. (eds.) (1996) *The Oxford textbook of psychiatry*, 3rd edn. Oxford University Press, Oxford, pp. 270–272.

6.6

a **True.** Also known as cardiomegalia glycogenica diffusa or acid maltase deficiency.

b **False.** Autosomal recessive disorder of protein metabolism.

c **True.** Also known as mucopolysaccharidosis type II.

d **False.** X-linked recessive.

e **False.** Autosomal dominant.

Puri, B. and Tyrer, P. (1992) *Sciences basic to psychiatry*. Churchill Livingstone, Edinburgh, pp. 158–161.

Questions

6.7

	[Certainty]		
In the study of genetic disorders	High	Med	Low
a DNA mutations are seldom substitutions.	...	...	...
b Both introns and exons code for genetic material.	...	...	...
c Junk DNA codes for stop commands.	...	...	...
d Translocation takes place on the ribosomes.	...	...	...
e Normal males have a single Barr body.	...	...	...

6.8

Long term, or secondary memory			
a Has an unlimited capacity.	...	...	...
b Is also known as eidetic imagery.	...	...	...
c For events is termed episodic memory.	...	...	...
d Information retrieval is hindered by repression of emotionally charged material.	...	...	...
e Forgetfulness is a result of storage failure.	...	...	...

6.9

Regarding measurement scales in psychology:			
a The Likert scale is a 10-point scale.	...	...	...
b The semantic differential scale has a low test–retest reliability but is easy to use.	...	...	...
c The Likert scale can lead to differing response patterns resulting in the same mean score.	...	...	...
d The Thurstone scale is a dichotomous scale indicating agreement/disagreement with presented statements.	...	...	...
e The semantic differential scale is a visual analogue scale.	...	...	...

Answers
6.7

a **False.** DNA mutations are most often substitutions.

b **False.** Introns do not code for genetic material.

c **False.** Junk DNA has no known function. Specific triplet sequences code for the stop and start commands along DNA.

d **False.** Translocation involves the breakage of a part of a chromosome and is a type of DNA mutation. Translation (formation of peptide chains from genetic code) takes place on ribosomes.

e **False.** This is also known as a chromatin body. The number of Barr bodies seen in a cell nuclei equates to the number of X chromosomes minus one. Normal males have no Barr body.

Puri, B. and Tyrer, P. (1992) *Sciences basic to psychiatry*. Churchill Livingstone, Edinburgh, pp. 146–151.

6.8

a **True.** This is theoretically true, although there are usually limitations on retrieval.

b **False.** Eidetic imagery is a photographic memory, seen in about 5% of children. A detailed visual image can be retained for over half a minute.

c **True.** This provides a continually changing and updated record of auto-biographical material. Semantic memory stores verbal information in terms of meaning rather than exact words.

d **True.** Negative emotions and anxiety hinder retrieval.

e **False.** Believed to be a result of retrieval failure. Said to explain hypnosis aided memory recovery and the 'tip of the tongue' phenomenon.

Puri, B. and Hall, A.D. (1998) *Revision notes in psychiatry* 1. Arnold, London, pp. 7–8.

6.9

a **False.** The Likert scale is a five-point scale indicating the level of agreement with presented statements.

b **False.** This bipolar visual analogue scale is easy to use and has good test–retest reliability. Positional response bias may occur.

c **True.** As can the Thurstone scale. However, the Likert scale has increased sensitivity and is easier to administer than the Thurstone scale.

d **True.** The presented statements are ranked, which can lead to bias.

e **True.**

Puri, B. and Hall, A.D. (1998) *Revision notes in psychiatry* 2. Arnold, London, p. 1.

Questions
6.10   [Certainty]

Attachment theory	High	Med	Low
a Is associated with the work of Winnicott.	...	...	...
b Gives a theoretical basis for grieving.	...	...	...
c Suggests early childhood experience is important for later mental health.	...	...	...
d Is not applicable to therapy with the elderly.	...	...	...
e Emphasizes the importance of internalising a secure 'good object'.	...	...	...

6.11
Examples of 'displacement activity' are

	High	Med	Low
a Drinking alcohol to excess.	...	...	...
b Scratching.	...	...	...
c Pacing up and down.	...	...	...
d Driving recklessly.	...	...	...
e Lighting a cigarette.	...	...	...

6.12
The following non-verbal behaviours can have communicative functions in groups:

	High	Med	Low
a Facilitators.	...	...	...
b Illustrators.	...	...	...
c Regulators.	...	...	...
d Adaptors.	...	...	...
e Emblems.	...	...	...

6.13
Characteristics of a profession include:

	High	Med	Low
a Ability to charge a fee.	...	...	...
b Possession of a monopoly in the field.	...	...	...
c Providing altruistic service.	...	...	...
d Not going on strike.	...	...	...
e Extended period of formal training and education.	...	...	...

Answers
6.10

    a **False.** This area is principally associated with the work of John Bowlby. Winnicott (a paediatrician, originally) wrote about child development and 'self psychology'.

    b **True.** Parkes postulated attachment theory as a basis for grief and loss.

    c **True.**

    d **False.** The cycle of attachment, loss, and grief continues throughout life.

    e **True.** It is said that an unavailable mother can interfere with normal internalization of a 'good object'.

Holmes, J. (1991) *Textbook of psychotherapy in psychiatric practice.* Churchill Livingstone, Edinburgh, pp. 21–22.

6.11

    a **False.**

    b **True.**

    c **True.**

    d **False.**

    e **True.**

Note: Displacement activity is an instinctive movement used as an outlet for energy bottled up when some action is blocked by a conflicting drive. It was observed initially by Konrad Lorenz in sticklebacks. Driving recklessly and drinking alcohol are not instinctive movements.

Weller, M. and Eysenck, M. (1991) *The scientific basis of psychiatry*, 2nd edn. Saunders, Philadelphia, pp. 449–450.

6.12

    a **False.** There is no such term.

    b **True.** These behaviours can supplement speech, e.g. pointing while explaining directions.

    c **True.** These are behaviours which control interactions, such as eye contact indicating who can speak.

    d **True.** Attempts to maintain self control such as fidgeting or scratching.

    e **True.** Signs which are complete on their own such as a 'thumbs up'.

Weller, M. and Eysenck, M. (1991) *The scientific basis of psychiatry*, 2nd edn. Saunders, Philadelphia, pp. 465–466.

6.13

    a **False.** Although professionals' fees tend to be higher!

    b **True.** The state should recognize the professional organization.

    c **True.** As well as adherence to a code of conduct.

    d **False.** However, going on strike is said to decrease professionalism.

    e **True.** Also, assessments of competence carried out by the profession.

Puri, B. and Hall, A.D. (1998) *Revision notes in psychiatry* 7. Arnold, London, pp 80–81.

Questions

6.14
[Certainty]

The following describe dysfunctional family relationships:

	High	Med	Low
a Enmeshed families.	...	...	...
b Engaged families.	...	...	...
c Triangulation.	...	...	...
d Non-ambiguous communication.	...	...	...
e Families which create myths.	...	...	...

6.15

Reported advantages ensuing from a sectorized community mental health service are

a Minimizing patients lost to follow-up.	...	...	...
b Preference by patients and relatives.	...	...	...
c Enhanced patient compliance with medication.	...	...	...
d Better training environment for staff.	...	...	...
e Improved primary care liaison potential.	...	...	...

6.16

The Brief Psychiatric Rating Scale (BPRS)

a Is a self-rating scale.	...	...	...
b Comprises 11 items on a 7-point scale.	...	...	...
c Is particularly suitable for patients with minor psychiatric illness.	...	...	...
d Has a low inter-rater reliability.	...	...	...
e Enables computer-aided diagnosis from the symptom profile and scores obtained.	...	...	...

Answers
6.14

a **True.** Individuals lack autonomy and self-identity. They are less able to respond to external cues or advice.

b **False.** Disengaged families, where there is a lack of family unity.

c **True.** A mixture of close and distant relationships, e.g. the father who forms a close attachment to the daughter and withdraws away from the mother.

d **False.** Ambiguous communication where there is incongruity between what is said and the way it is expressed.

e **True.** Almost to the point of delusion, e.g. that there is nothing wrong with the family relationship.

Tantum, D. and Birchwood, M. (eds.) (1994) *Seminars in psychology and the social sciences.* Gaskell, London, pp. 270–272.

6.15

a **True.** Running *pari passu* with a defined responsibility for each patient requiring a service.

b **True.** Also greater facilities for home treatment and day care services.

c **False.** This might be a consequence of (a) but sectorization has no direct impact on this for the individual patient.

d **False.** Although the identity of staff with the locality is improved and optimizing the system might lead to improved morale.

e **True.** With better interagency working, and a supposedly integrated health, social, and voluntary service provision.

Bhugra, D. and Leff, J. (eds.) (1993) *Principles of social psychiatry.* Blackwell, Oxford, pp. 479–485.

6.16

a **False.** The BPRS is a scale for rating severity of symptoms and signs of psychiatric disturbance. It is completed by an observer conducting a semi-structured interview. Ratings are based on observation and patients' verbal report.

b **True.**

c **False.** It is unsuitable for patients with minor psychiatric illness.

d **False.** The inter-rater reliability is satisfactory in itself and can be improved further by jointly 2 observers rating and average the score.

e **True.**

Kendell, R.E. and Zealley, A.K. (eds.) (1993) *Companion to psychiatric studies*, 5th edn. Churchill Livingstone, Edinburgh, p. 173.

Questions
6.17
[Certainty]

	High	Med	Low
Difficulties associated with meta-analysis include			
a Non-inclusion of negative result studies.	...	...	...
b Adequate and acceptable inclusion criteria for varying studies.	...	...	...
c Applying results to a specific population from trials conducted on differing populations.	...	...	...
d Not all individuals have reached the study event during the time interval studied.	...	...	...
e A high chance of a type II error.	...	...	...

6.18
The following are mental or behavioural disorders specified in ICD 10:

	High	Med	Low
a Nose picking.	...	...	...
b Satyriasis.	...	...	...
c Pica.	...	...	...
d Culture shock.	...	...	...
e Aerophagy.	...	...	...

6.19
Peptide neurotransmitters

	High	Med	Low
a Have a relatively low affinity for their receptors.	...	...	...
b Are active in lower concentrations than classical transmitters.	...	...	...
c Include gastrin.	...	...	...
d Are synthesized at a faster rate than classical neurotransmitters in the nerve terminals.	...	...	...
e Have a higher molecular weight than classical neurotransmitters.	...	...	...

Answers
6.17

a **True.** Significant results are more likely to be published than non-significant ones, and researchers may be less likely to write up negative result studies.

b **True.** Arriving at selection criteria which are stringent and yet inclusive is difficult.

c **True.** Different study centres may differ in important ways diminishing the validity of combining data and generalizing results.

d **False.** This statement applies to the technique of survival analysis.

e **False.** A type II error is concerned with wrongly accepting a false null hypothesis. Meta-analysis should increase power by pooling data.

Puri, B. and Hall, A.D. (1998) *Revision notes in psychiatry* 6. Arnold, London, pp. 67–68.

6.18

a **True.** Perhaps surprisingly this is coded as a disorder of childhood and adolescence (F98.8).

b **True.** This is a disorder of excessive sexual drive, synonymous with nymphomania and coded F52.7, said to occur in men and women during late teenage or early adult life.

c **True.** Specified in both adults (F50.8—non-organic origin) and children (F98.3) Can be defined as the persistent eating of non-nutritive substances.

d **True.** As well as being the title of a book by Alvin Toffler, this is an adjustment disorder with affective symptoms (F43.28).

e **True.** This is a neurotic somatoform disorder (F45.31) of the upper gastrointestinal tract, meaning to 'swallow air'.

World Health Organization (1992) *Tenth revision of the International Classification of Disease (ICD 10)*. WHO, Geneva.

6.19

a **False.** They have a high affinity for their receptors.

b **True.**

c **True.**

d **False.** They are synthesized at a slower rate.

e **True.** Peptides have a higher potency than classical neurotransmitters, and so are effective at lower concentrations. Both classical and peptide transmitters have a high affinity for their receptors. There are many peptides now known to be neurotransmitters including somatostatin, ACTH, gastrin, bombesin, and CCK. They generally have a much higher molecular weight than classical transmitters.

Leonard, B.F. (1997) *Fundamentals of psychopharmacology*. Wiley, New York, pp. 21–24.

Questions
6.20
[Certainty]

Correct pairings of drug and group include:	High	Med	Low
a Chlormethiazole—azaspirodecanedione.	...	...	...
b Cyclizine—cyclopyrrolone.	...	...	...
c Triazolam—benzodiazepine.	...	...	...
d Buspirone—propanediol.	...	...	...
e Zopiclone—antihistamine.	...	...	...

6.21
Concerning clozapine:

	High	Med	Low
a Hepatic metabolites include norclozapine.	...	...	...
b Metabolism involves the cytochrome p450 system.	...	...	...
c Smoking cigarettes can raise clozapine levels.	...	...	...
d Carbamazepine may be useful in treating clozapine induced seizures.	...	...	...
e Serotonin re-uptake inhibitor (SSRI) antidepressants increase clozapine levels.	...	...	...

6.22
Glycine

	High	Med	Low
a Is excitatory in nature.	...	...	...
b Is found mostly in the spinal cord.	...	...	...
c Can be biosynthesized from alanine.	...	...	...
d Receptors are blocked by strychnine.	...	...	...
e Release at neurones may be inhibited by tetanus toxin.	...	...	...

6.23
Glucocorticoids

	High	Med	Low
a Given in high doses cause psychiatric disorder in approximately 20% of patients.	...	...	...
b Are known to be neurotoxic to the hippocampus	...	...	...
c Directly inhibit the secretion of ACTH at the level of the hypothalamus.	...	...	...
d If non-suppressed by dexamethasone are a robust indicator of prognosis in depression.	...	...	...
e If exogenous, are more likely to cause elevation of the mood than if there is excessive endogenous secretion.	...	...	...

Answers
6.20

    a **False.** Chlormethiazole—propanediol.
    b **False.** Cyclizine—antihistamine.
    c **True.**
    d **False.** Buspirone—azaspirodecanedione.
    e **False.** Zopiclone—cyclopyrrolone.

Puri, B. and Tyrer, P. (1992) *Sciences basic to psychiatry*. Churchill Livingstone, Edinburgh, pp. 133–134.

6.21

    a **True.**
    b **True.**
    c **False.** This can have the reverse effect. There is a case report of a man who developed clozapine induced seizures on stopping smoking!
    d **False.** A potentially dangerous combination due to the increased risk of neutropenia.
    e **True.** Therefore should be used with caution.

Taylor, D. (1997) Pharmacokinetic interactions involving clozapine. *British Journal of Psychiatry* 171, 109–112.

6.22

    a **False.** An inhibitory amino acid neurotransmitter.
    b **True.**
    c **False.** From serine via serine hyrdroxymethylase.
    d **True.**
    e **False.** Release can be induced by tetanus toxin.

Puri, B. and Tyrer, P. (1992) *Sciences basic to psychiatry*. Churchill Livingstone, Edinburgh, p. 94.

6.23

    a **True.** Disturbance of mood, sleep, and cognition are common when normal subjects are given glucocorticoids. This may be severe enough to cause psychiatric disorder.
    b **True.** The hippocampus is the main site of feedback control for the hypothalamo–pituitary–adrenal axis with many glucocorticoid receptors.
    c **False.** ACTH is secreted by the pituitary and so reduction of ACTH secretion by the hypothalamus is indirect.
    d **True.** Non-suppression of cortisol secretion after dexamethasone is a good indicator of poor prognosis.
    e **True.** Depression rather than elation is common in Cushing's syndrome, whereas exogenous steroids leads to elation more frequently.

Mitchell, A. and O'Keane, V. (1998) Steroids and depression: glucocorticoid steroids affect behaviour and mood. *British Medical Journal* 316, 244–245.

Questions
6.24

	[Certainty]		
Synaptic transmission	High	Med	Low
a Can occur between several different areas of the surface of a neuron.	...	...	...
b Is quickest if the transmission involves chemical neurotransmitters.	...	...	...
c Can be bi-directional in the human nervous system.	...	...	...
d Is more often by chemical than electrical means.	...	...	...
e Occurs across a distance of approximately 25 μm.	...	...	...

6.25

In normal adult sleep			
a Stages 2, 3, and 4 combined give a measurement of the total slow wave sleep.	...	...	...
b K complexes are seen in stage 1.	...	...	...
c REM sleep occupies nearly 50% of sleep.	...	...	...
d θ waves on the EEG are characteristic of stage 3.	...	...	...
e Slow wave sleep aids cerebral restitution.	...	...	...

Answers
6.24

a **True.** Synapses can be axo-dendritic, dendro-dendritic, axo-somatic, and somato-somatic.

b **False.** Electrical transmission is quicker than chemical.

c **True.**

d **True.** Chemical synapses are more common in humans.

e **False.** The gap across a synaptic cleft is closer to 25 nm (i.e. 1000 times smaller).

Puri, B. and Tyrer, P. (1992) *Sciences basic to psychiatry*. Churchill Livingstone, Edinburgh, pp. 25–28.

6.25

a **False.** Stages 3 and 4 give total deep or slow wave sleep.

b **False.** K complexes are characteristic of stage 2 sleep.

c **False.** In the adult, REM sleep occurs 4–5 times per night and lasts in total about 90 minutes (about 20–25%). On the EEG, low voltage mixed frequency patterns are seen, with saw-tooth waves. About 50% of infantile sleep is REM.

d **False.** θ waves are seen in stage 2, whereas δ waves are observed in stages 3 and 4.

e **True.** However, the exact function of both REM and deep sleep is unknown.

Cowen, P.J. (1997) *Depression and sleep*. Martin Dunitz, London, pp. 1–7.

Questions

Clinical

6.26   [Certainty]

In Huntington's disease	High	Med	Low
a The pattern of inheritance is autosomal dominant with incomplete penetrance.	...	...	...
b Language function is relatively spared in the early stages.	...	...	...
c Depletion of glutamate is implicated in the aetiology.	...	...	...
d The phenomena of 'anticipation' is likely.	...	...	...
e Preclinical testing should be performed in all 'at risk' people.	...	...	...

6.27

Lewy body disease/dementia (LBD)			
a Is the second most common type of degenerative pathology in demented patients.	...	...	...
b Pathology is almost identical to Parkinson's disease.	...	...	...
c Commonly coexists with Alzheimers's disease pathology.	...	...	...
d More commonly affects women than men.	...	...	...
e Patients show particular impairment in visuospatial tests.	...	...	...

Answers

Clinical

6.26

a **False.** Complete penetrance.

b **True.** It cause a subcortical dementia and involuntary and voluntary move-ment disorders with choreoathetosis, bradykinesia, and disrupted gait and dexterity. Early cognitive deficits observed are impaired attention, problem solving and memory.

c **False.** Neural degeneration begins in the striatum, where neurones contain-ing GABA and GABA's synthesizing enzyme, glutamic acid decarboxylase, are depleted.

d **True.** The gene has been located at the tip of the short arm of chromosome 4. In affected cases a part of the gene is expanded and shows trinucleotide repeats. These repeat sequences tend to increase in successive generations with the longest segments being found in juvenile onset or paternal transmission cases ('anticipation').

e **False.** The development of an accurate preclinical test has important ethical considerations. People at risk should be counselled as to the implications of a positive test, and their wishes respected should they not wish to go ahead with testing.

Purdon, S.E., Mohr, E., Ilivitsky, V., *et al.* (1994) Huntington's disease: pathogenesis, diag-nosis and treatment (review). *Journal of Psychiatry and Neuroscience* 19(5), 359–367.

6.27

a **True.** Lewy bodies have been demonstrated in 15–25% of cases of dementia in several autopsy studies.

b **False.** The pathology is far more widespread in LBD and includes areas such as the hippocampus, temporal lobes and neocortex. They are also more numerous.

c **True.**

d **False.** Men are more commonly affected.

e **True.** As compared with Alzheimer's patients with a similar degree of dementia.

McKeith, I.G., Galasko, D., Wilcock, G.K., *et al.* (1995) Lewy body dementia-diagnosis and treatment. *British Journal of Psychiatry* 167, 709–718.

Questions
6.28

	[Certainty]		
Dementia of frontal lobe type	High	Med	Low
a Is a common subtype of dementia.	...	...	...
b Is associated with the disappearance of frontal release reflexes.	...	...	...
c Results in early impairment of verbal fluency.	...	...	...
d Is synonymous with Pick's disease.	...	...	...
e Is usually of insidious onset.	...	...	...

6.29

Following head injury

a Retrograde amnesia is more useful than post-traumatic amnesia (PTA) in assessing prognosis.	...	...	...
b Those with a PTA of less than 1 hour will usually be back at work within 1 month of the injury.	...	...	...
c The length of PTA is linked with personality change.	...	...	...
d The onset of dementia is common when the injury is severe.	...	...	...
e Post-traumatic epilepsy develops in about 10% of closed head injuries.	...	...	...

6.30

The central nervous system effects of alcohol include:

a Central pontine myelinosis.	...	...	...
b VIth nerve palsy.	...	...	...
c Degeneration of the corpus callosum.	...	...	...
d Truncal cerebellar ataxia.	...	...	...
e Progressive supranuclear palsy.	...	...	...

Answers

6.28

    a **True.** Dementia of frontal lobe type (DFT) is relatively common, accounting for 10–20% of all cases of dementia.

    b **False.** Primitive reflexes such as grasp, pout, palmomental reflexes reappear.

    c **True.** Poor verbal fluency is one of the most sensitive tests.

    d **False.** Pick's disease is one of the DFT, and constitutes about 2.5% of all dementias.

    e **True.** The onset of DFT is insidious, with personality change, disinhibition, apathy, and empty or fatuous euphoria being common early features.

Orrell, M. W. and Sahakian, B. J. (1991) Dementia of the frontal lobe type. *Psychological Medicine* 21, 553–556.

6.29

    a **False.** PTA may be used as an index of severity.

    b **True.** With PTA of less than 1 day patients may be back to work within 2 months.

    c **True.** And also to intellectual impairment, euphoria, and aspects of frontal lobe syndrome.

    d **False.** Relative rarity of enduring, profound dementia even after severe injuries.

    e **False.** Usually less than 5%. If the dura mater is penetrated this rises to 30%.

Lishman, W.A. (1998) *Organic Psychiatry* , 3rd edn. Blackwell Science, Oxford, pp. 171–177.

6.30

    a **True.** Central pontine myelinosis is thought to be due to rapid shifts in sodium associated with rehydration.

    b **True.** VIth nerve palsy may be due to Wernicke's encephalopathy, trauma, central pontine myelinosis, or neuropathy.

    c **True.** Marchiafava–Bignami syndrome is a form of degeneration of the corpus callosum.

    d **True.** Cerebellar damage is a direct toxic effect, and tends to be truncal rather than distal.

    e **False.** Progressive supranuclear palsy (or Steele–Richardson–Olszewski syndrome) is a rare degenerative disorder.

Note: The cerebral consequences of alcohol abuse are as much neuropsychological as neurological, and can be helpfully divided into those of acute intoxication; withdrawal; and chronic abuse.

Lishman, W.A. (1998) *Organic psychiatry*, 3rd edn. Blackwell Science, Oxford, pp. 585–587.

Questions
6.31

Reboxetine	[Certainty]		
	High	Med	Low
a Is a selective inhibitor of serotonin re-uptake.	...	...	...
b Causes insomnia.	...	...	...
c Causes paraesthesia.	...	...	...
d Can be started immediately after a monoamine oxidase inhibitor (MAOI) is discontinued.	...	...	...
e Can be given safely to breast-feeding mothers.	...	...	...

6.32

Antipsychotics			
a In high doses have been implicated in a number of sudden deaths in psychiatric patients.	...	...	...
b Have a positive inotropic effect.	...	...	...
c In high doses show superior effectiveness than standard doses in treatment-resistant patients.	...	...	...
d Effectively block 70–90% of dopamine receptors at the equivalent of modest doses of chlorpromazine, e.g. 300–400 mg.	...	...	...
e Such as chlorpromazine have a British National Formulary advisory maximum daily dose of 1500 mg.	...	...	...

6.33

The following factors may make a patient less likely to fit during a course of ECT:

a Male sex.	...	...	...
b Low blood oxygen saturation.	...	...	...
c Current use of theophylline.	...	...	...
d Paget's disease.	...	...	...
e Baldness.	...	...	...

6.34

The following help differentiate bereavement from a depressive episode:

a Suicidal ideation.	...	...	...
b Marked psychomotor retardation.	...	...	...
c Morbid preoccupation with worthlessness.	...	...	...
d Reduced latency of verbal response.	...	...	...
e Anhedonia.	...	...	...

Answers

6.31

a **False.** It is a selective inhibitor of noradrenaline re-uptake.

b **True.**

c **True.**

d **False.** Have to wait at least 2 weeks. Similarly, have to wait 1 week after discontinuing reboxetine before being able to start an MAOI.

e **False.** It is a new drug and little information is available on this subject. The manufacturer advises not giving the drug to mothers who are breast-feeding.

British National Formulary, Section 4.3.4 and Appendix 1 and 5.

6.32

a **True.**

b **False.** A negative inotropic effect of reducing cardiac output and lowering of blood pressure.

c **False.** Controlled trials have not shown this to be true.

d **True.** This can be demonstrated using positron emission tomography (PET).

e **False.** 1000 mg. Increasing the dose beyond this limit requires careful consideration of clinical, social, and psychological variables, and a careful analysis of the potential risks and benefits.

Thompson, C. (1994) The use of high-dose antipsychotic medication. *British Journal of Psychiatry* 164, 448–458.

6.33

a **True.** Males have higher seizure threshold than females.

b **True.** Hence the use of hyperventilation to increase the likelihood of a seizure.

c **False.** This lowers the threshold, as does caffeine.

d **True.** This condition is characterized by thickening of bones including the cranium.

e **True.** Due to impaired contact with electrodes.

Locke, T. (1994) Advances in the practice of ECT. *Advances in Psychiatric Treatment* 1, 47–56.

6.34

a **False.**

b **True.** Also, guilt about things other than actions taken or not taken at the time of the loss.

c **True.** Thoughts of death, other than the survivor feeling they also should have died, or would be better off dead, also discriminate.

d **False.** Long pauses in speech can be seen in both.

e **False.**

Note: A DSM IV diagnosis of major depressive disorder is generally not given unless symptoms are still present 2 months after the loss. Hallucinatory experiences other than hearing the voice of, or transiently seeing the image of the deceased are not characteristic of bereavement.

Puri, B.K. and Hall, A.D. (1998) *Revision notes in psychiatry* 5. Arnold, London, p. 43.

Questions
6.35

[Certainty]

Regarding deliberate self harm (DSH)

	High	Med	Low
a Rates are increasing in young females in the UK.	...	...	...
b Rates in the UK are among the highest in Europe.	...	...	...
c Repetition rate is approximately 30% within one year.	...	...	...
d Rates in young men are stable.	...	...	...
e It has a strong association with substance abuse in young men.	...	...	...

6.36

Adolescents with anorexia nervosa

a Have a good outcome in approximately 50 % of cases.	...	...	...
b Should have a programme aimed at gaining 3–4 kg per week.	...	...	...
c If female, may have a normal menstrual cycle.	...	...	...
d Always have an intense fear of gaining weight or becoming fat.	...	...	...
e Have a long-term suicide rate of approximately 10–15%.	...	...	...

6.37

The following are true of attention deficit hyperactivity disorder (ADHD):

a Symptoms rarely persist into adult life.	...	...	...
b There is an increased prevalence of ADHD in first degree relatives of childhood ADHD probands.	...	...	...
c Magnetic resonance imaging has demonstrated structural cerebellar abnormalities.	...	...	...
d In adults it may be difficult to distinguish from personality disorder.	...	...	...
e In adults with ADHD, treatment with amphetamines has produced beneficial effects in the majority.	...	...	...

Answers
6.35

    a **True.** There has been a gradual increase in recent years.

    b **True.**

    c **False.** The repetition rate in the UK is approximately 15% within one year.

    d **False.** There has been a marked increase in the rate of deliberate self-harm in young men in recent years.

    e **True.**

Note: There appears to have been a substantial increase in the rate of DSH in the UK over the last few years. The increase is particularly marked in young men and is associated with substance abuse. In the study cited, rates of repetition were found to be increasing and paracetamol was used in half of all episodes of DSH. This increase in DSH has important implications for the likely suicide rate, and Health of the Nation targets for reductions.

Hawton, K., Fagg, J., Simkin, S., *et al*. (1997) Trends in deliberate self harm in Oxford 1985–1995. *British Journal of Psychiatry* 171, 556–560.

6.36

    a **True.**

    b **False.** A more accurate figure would be 0.5–1 kg per week.

    c **False.** The DSM IV diagnostic criteria specify that in postmenarcheal females a diagnosis is made only if amenorrheac.

    d **True.** This is a diagnostic criterion.

    e **False.** Approximately 5%.

Black, D. and Cottrell, D. (eds.) (1993) *Seminars in child and adolescent psychiatry*. Gaskell, London, pp. 175–178.

6.37

    a **False.** Some follow-up studies have shown almost one quarter at age 16–23 continue to meet the criteria for diagnosis compared with 3% of controls. Approximately 0.5–1% of the young adult population have associated problems.

    b **True.**

    c **False.**

    d **True.** Including intermittent explosive behaviour, inattention, impulsivity, and personal disorganization.

    e **False.** Studies have concluded that up to one quarter may show some improvement.

Toone, B.K. and Van der Linden, G.J.H. (1997) Attention deficit hyperactivity disorder in adults. *British Journal of Psychiatry* 170, 489–491.

Questions
6.38

	[Certainty]		
Stammering	High	Med	Low
a Is a disturbance of the rhythm and fluency of speech.	...	...	...
b Is equally common in boys and girls.	...	...	...
c Affects 1 in 20 children aged 5.	...	...	...
d Is usually associated with a psychiatric disorder.	...	...	...
e Is best treated with psychotherapy and behavioural therapy.	...	...	...

6.39

The following are true of psychopathy:

a A high degree of impulsivity is usually present.	...	...	...
b Family studies have indicated a link with attention deficit hyperactivity disorder.	...	...	...
c Twin studies have not shown a significant genetic component.	...	...	...
d Possessing XYY chromosomes has been demonstrated to be directly linked with aggressive behaviour.	...	...	...
e A link with low 5HT activity has been postulated.	...	...	...

6.40

Rape

a Refers only to completed vaginal intercourse.	...	...	...
b Results in 75% of victims developing a chronic psychiatric disorder.	...	...	...
c Victims commonly experience sexual dysfunction.	...	...	...
d Complicated by post-traumatic stress disorder (PTSD) is predicted by an initial rapid resolution of symptoms within the first 2 weeks.	...	...	...
e Victims, like other trauma victims, have shown good responses to eye-movement desensitization and reprocessing (EMDR).	...	...	...

Answers

6.38

  a **True.**

  b **False.** It is four times as common in boys.

  c **False.** It affects approximately 1% of children at school entry.

  d **False.** It can cause embarrassment and distress but is not usually associated with a psychiatric disorder.

  e **False.** The usual treatment is speech therapy.

Gelder, M., Gath, D., Mayou, R., and Cowen, P. (eds.) (1996) *The Oxford textbook of psychiatry*, 3rd edn. Oxford University Press, Oxford, p. 710.

6.39

  a **True.**

  b **True.** Impulsivity is linked to some of the core features of psychopathy, including inability to delay gratification and lack of feeling for others.

  c **False.** Concordance rates of 51% in monozygotic and 22% in dizygotic twins have been shown.

  d **False.**

  e **True.**

Dolan, M. (1994) Psychopathy: a neurobiological perspective. *British Journal of Psychiatry* 165, 151–160.

6.40

  a **False.** The legal definition of rape is narrower than the social one. The Criminal Justice and Public Order Act 1994 now recognize the existence of male rape victims by including anal as well as vaginal penetration within its definition.

  b **False.** The majority do not develop a chronic psychiatric disorder.

  c **True.** Usually reported as decreased enjoyment due to re-experiencing symptoms and flashbacks.

  d **False.** An initial rapid resolution of symptoms predicts a good prognosis. Bad prognostic factors include completed rape, physical injury, and perception of life threat during the attack.

  e **True.** Although the evidence is still preliminary.

Mezey, G.C. (1997) Treatment of rape victims. *Advances in Psychiatric Treatment*, 3, 197–203.

Questions
6.41

Transexualism

	High	Med	Low
a Is a recognized diagnosis according to ICD 10.	...	...	...
b Includes a desire to live and be accepted as a member of the opposite sex.	...	...	...
c Involves sexual excitement from wearing clothes of the opposite sex.	...	...	...
d Is usually accompanied by a genetic or sex chromosomal abnormality.	...	...	...
e May be accompanied by a diagnosis of schizophrenia.	...	...	...

6.42

Regarding dysthymia:

a The majority of clinical cases go on to develop a major depression.	...	...	...
b A depressive illness occurring in a dysthymia sufferer is known as double depression.	...	...	...
c Kraepelin was the first to give a clinical description of the syndrome.	...	...	...
d Anti-depressants have been proposed as the mainstay of treatment.	...	...	...
e The highest comorbidity is with eating disorders.	...	...	...

6.43

In the assessment of risk and dangerousness

a Psychiatrists tend to under-predict dangerousness.	...	...	...
b Age, gender, and social class are among the best predictors of violence.	...	...	...
c Serious violence during an ictal phenomenon is rare.	...	...	...
d Psychiatric disorder is not a significant contributor towards dangerousness.	...	...	...
e It is easier to assess dangerousness in those with personality disorder compared to those with a mental illness.	...	...	...

Answers
6.41

    a **True.**

    b **True.** Usually accompanied by a sense of discomfort of one's anatomic sex and a wish to have hormonal treatment or surgery to transform one's body to the preferred sex.

    c **False.** The wearing of clothes of the opposite sex principally to obtain sexual excitement is known as fetishistic transvestism (ICD 10, F65.1).

    d **False.** These are exclusion criteria for a diagnosis according to ICD 10.

    e **False.** Again this is an exclusion criteria for a diagnosis according to ICD 10.

World Health Organization (1992) *Tenth revision of the International Classification of Disease (ICD 10).* WHO, Geneva, pp. 215–218.

6.42

    a **True.**

    b **True.**

    c **False.** Kahlbaum.

    d **True.** Tricyclics, serotonin re-uptake inhibitors and reversible inhibitors of monoamine oxidase have been shown to be 2–3.75 times more effective than placebo.

    e **False.** Major depression, followed by panic disorder. Substance abuse is also a relatively frequent finding.

WPA Dysthymia working group. (1995) Dysthymia in clinical practice. *British Journal of Psychiatry* **166**, 174–183.

6.43

    a **False.** Psychiatrists tend to over-predict dangerousness. Of every three disordered patients predicted to be violent, only one will go on to commit a violent act.

    b **True.** As is the case for the non-disordered population.

    c **True.**

    d **True.** Although certain specific psychiatric symptoms (e.g. delusional jealousy) can be dangerous.

    e **False.** The reverse is true.

Kendell, R.E. and Zealley, A.K. (eds.) (1993) *Companion to psychiatric studies*, 5th edn. Churchill Livingstone, Edinburgh, pp. 804–807.

Questions
6.44

	[Certainty]		
Essential issues to be addressed in a psychiatric court report include:	High	Med	Low
a Prognosis.	...	...	...
b Attitude to the alleged offence.	...	...	...
c Previous criminological history.	...	...	...
d Financial state of defendant.	...	...	...
e Mental state at the time of interview.	...	...	...

6.45

The following causes of mortality are greater in schizophrenia compared to the general population:			
a Natural causes.	...	...	...
b Accidents.	...	...	...
c Suicide.	...	...	...
d Homicide.	...	...	...
e Undetermined deaths.	...	...	...

6.46

High expressed emotion by relatives			
a Is characterized by marital schism.	...	...	...
b Is characterized by triangulation.	...	...	...
c Leads to an increased risk of relapse in schizophrenia which is protected by being on antipsychotics.	...	...	...
d Is less common in western countries compared to developing countries.	...	...	...
e Leads to a worse overall prognosis in schizophrenia.	...	...	...

6.47

Munchausen syndrome by proxy			
a Was first described by a psychiatrist called Meadow.	...	...	...
b Has epilepsy as the most common illness invented by mothers for their children.	...	...	...
c Is associated with psychological overdependence of the child on the mother.	...	...	...
d May be understood by the defence mechanism of sublimation.	...	...	...
e Is characterized by psychotic illness in the mother in around 35% of cases.	...	...	...

Answers
6.44

a **False.** This is not always essential, but may be given where relevant. Also, some justifiable opinion on future risk to self or others may be requested or supplied.

b **True.** It is important to record the defendant's own account of his or her actions and state of mind at the time of offence(s).

c **False.** This is usually provided.

d **False.** Not always relevant.

e **True.** If there is no detectable mental disorder this may be very brief.

Chiswick, D. and Cope R. (eds.) (1995) *Seminars in forensic psychiatry*. Gaskell, London, pp. 139–143.

6.45

a **False.** 80% of schizophrenia sufferers die from natural causes compared to 97% of the general population.

b **True.** Twice the rate of the general population.

c **True.** The largest single cause of the excess mortality in schizophrenia.

d **True.**

e **True.** This code is used if there is insufficient evidence to decide the cause of death.

Brown, S. (1997) Excess mortality in schizophrenia. *British Journal of Psychiatry* 171, 502–508.

6.46

a **False.**

b **False.** Features of high expressed emotion include critical comments, hostility, and over-involvement.

c **True.** This appears to be related to the amount of time the schizophrenic patient is in contact with the high expressed emotion from relatives.

d **False.** More common in western countries.

e **True.** The balance between over- and under-stimulation in schizophrenia is complex. It appears that excessive stimulation precipitates a relapse with positive symptoms and understimulation leads to worsening of negative symptoms.

Gelder, M., Gath, D., Mayou, R., and Cowen, P. (eds.) (1996) *The Oxford textbook of psychiatry*, 3rd edn. Oxford University Press, Oxford, pp. 284–285.

6.47

a **False.** A paediatrician. The child is usually brought to the attention of medical specialties prior to the diagnosis being considered.

b **True.**

c **False.** Overdependence of the mother on the child.

d **False.** Projective identification.

e **False.** Psychotic illness is relatively rare.

Bools, C. (1996) Factitious illness by proxy. *British Journal of Psychiatry* 169, 268–275.

Questions
6.48

	[Certainty]		
Abreaction	High	Med	Low
a Is the unrestrained expression of emotion.	...	...	...
b Often leads to the temporary relief of mental disorder.	...	...	...
c Is an established part of religious healing.	...	...	...
d Was used during wartime to bring rapid relief to soldiers suffering from anxiety.	...	...	...
e Is facilitated by sedative intravenous drugs.	...	...	...

6.49

Characteristic defences mechanisms used by patients with borderline personality disorder are

a Displacement.	...	...	...
b Splitting.	...	...	...
c Identification with the aggressor.	...	...	...
d Projective identification.	...	...	...
e Idealization.	...	...	...

Answers
6.48

a **True.** The method is said to be of value in the investigation and treatment of acute neuroses caused by stress.

b **True.**

c **True.**

d **True.** Thereby enabling soldiers to be returned to the front line.

e **True.** Abreaction can be facilitated by drugs such as intravenous barbiturates as well as by more diverse psychological techniques such as psychodrama.

Note: Abreaction was used in the past as a therapeutic manoeuvre in psychotherapy. It is used less often now. The term 'drug-assisted interview' is preferred to describe the technique, which is adjunctive to the investigation of patients who are otherwise inaccessible. Abreaction may lead to the discovery of new clinical information, although this is controversial with regard to the recovery of memories of childhood sexual abuse.

Gelder, M., Gath, D., Mayou, R., and Cowen, P. (eds.) (1996) *The Oxford textbook of psychiatry*, 3rd edn. Oxford University Press, Oxford, pp. 643.

Patrick, M. and Howells, R. (1990) Barbiturate assisted interviews in modern clinical practice. *Psychological Medicine* 20, 763–765.

6.49

a **False.**

b **True.**

c **False.**

d **True.**

e **True.**

Note: According to Otto Kernberg (one of the principal workers in this area) people with borderline personality disorders make excessive use of primitive defence mechanisms such as 'splitting' with omnipotence and devaluation, 'projective identification', primitive 'idealization', and some forms of 'denial'. The excessive use of these mechanisms or their failure may lead to disorder or psychiatric symptoms.

Bateman, A. (1991) Borderline personality disorder. In *Psychotherapy in psychiatric practice*, ed. J. Holmes. Churchill Livingstone, Edinburgh, pp. 335–337.

Questions
6.50
[Certainty]

According to Bloch and Crouch therapeutic factors in group psychotherapy include:

	High	Med	Low
a Acting out.	...	...	...
b Catharsis.	...	...	...
c Self-disclosure.	...	...	...
d Universality.	...	...	...
e Interpretation of transference.	...	...	...

Answers
6.50

   a **False.** Acting out generally refers to a pathological event whereby psychological conflicts are enacted outside the confines of the therapeutic group.

   b **True.** The experience of relief through the expression of feelings.

   c **True.**

   d **True.** The realization that one's problems are not unique.

   e **False.** Although this may occur it is not one of their therapeutic factors.

Note: Bloch and Crouch list 10 therapeutic factors—universality, acceptance, altruism, guidance, instillation of hope, catharsis, self-disclosure, interpersonal learning, vicarious learning, and self-understanding. A therapeutic factor is defined as 'an element of group therapy that contributes to the improvement in a patient's condition and is a function of the actions of the group therapist, the other group members and the patient himself'.

Hobbs, M. (1991) Group processes in psychiatry. In *Textbook of psychotherapy in psychiatric practice*, ed. J. Holmes, Churchill Livingstone, Edinburgh, pp. 62–64.

Questions by subject

Page numbers in brackets

Basic sciences

Genetics: 1.1 (1); 2.8 (37), 2.9 (37); 3.7 (71), 3.8 (71); 4.11 (105); 5.17 (139); 6.6 (163), 6.7 (165)

Neuroanatomy and neuropathology: 1.1 (1), 1.2 (1), 1.3 (1), 1.12 (7), 1.13 (9), 1.14 (9); 2.10 (37), 2.11 (37), 2.23 (45), 2.24 (47), 2.25 (47); 3.9 (71), 3.10 (73), 3.11 (73), 3.12 (73), 3.13 (75), 3.14 (75); 4.6 (101), 4.7 (103), 4.8 (103), 4.9 (103), 4.10 (103); 5.1 (129), 5.2 (129), 5.3 (129), 5.4 (131), 5.5 (131), 5.6 (131); 6.1 (161), 6.2 (161), 6.3 (161), 6.4 (163), 6.5 (163)

Neurochemistry, neuropharmacology, and neuroendocrinology: 1.15 (9), 1.16 (11), 1.17 (11), 1.18 (11), 1.21 (13); 2.4 (35), 2.5 (35), 2.6 (35), 2.7 (35); 3.7 (71), 3.15 (75), 3.16 (77), 3.17 (77), 3.18 (77), 3.19 (79), 3.20 (79); 4.11 (105), 4.12 (105), 4.13 (105), 4.14 (105), 4.15 (107), 4.18 109); 5.14 (137), 5.15 (137), 5.16 (137), 5.21 (141); 6.19 (171), 6.20 (173), 6.21 (173), 6.22 (173), 6.23 (173)

Neurophysiology: 1.19 (13), 1.20 (13); 2.12 (39), 2.13 (39), 2.14 (39), 2.15 (41); 3.20 (79), 3.21 (79), 3.22 (79); 4.16 (107), 4.17 (107); 5.18 (139), 5.19 (139), 5.20 (141); 6.24 (175), 6.25 (175)

Psychology and social sciences: 1.4 (3), 1.5 (3), 1.6 (3), 1.22 (13), 1.23 (15), 1.24 (15), 1.25 (15); 2.3 (33), 2.16 (41), 2.17 (41), 2.18 (43), 2.19 (43), 2.20 (43), 2.21 (45), 2.22 (45); 3.4 (69), 3.5 (69), 3.6 (69), 3.23 (81), 3.24 (81), 3.25 (81); 4.19 (109), 4.20 (109), 4.21 (111), 4.22 (111), 4.23 (111), 4.24 (113), 4.25 (113); 5.7 (133), 5.8 (133), 5.9 (133), 5.22 (141), 5.23 (141), 5.24 (143), 5.25 (143); 6.8 (165), 6.9 (165), 6.10 (167), 6.11 (167), 6.12 (167), 6.13 (167), 6.14 (169), 6.15 (169)

Clinical